Cross-Cultural Caring
A Handbook for Health Professionals in Western Canada

As western Canada's ethnic population increases, health care and social service workers are recognizing the importance of their being more aware of the particular needs of their ethnic patients in order to provide culturally sensitive and effective treatment programs.

This handbook describes several recent immigrant groups in western Canada, among them Vietnamese, South and Southeast Asians, Chinese, Japanese, Central Americans, West Indians, and Iranians. It is unique in its approach, as it provides information not only about the health beliefs and practices of these communities but also about the social context of each group.

Each chapter describes one particular ethnic group and discusses its attitudes towards such issues as childbirth, mental illness, dental care, hospitalization, and death. Information is also given on the level of health care, the religion, education, and political system in the home country, as well as on the reasons for emigrating and problems of adjusting to life in Canada. The authors, who are themselves members of the communities they describe, work in a wide variety of health-related fields. The information they provide reflects the kinds of questions professionals ask about these immigrant groups.

The final chapter offers specific guidelines for cultural assessment, including strategies for negotiating a plan of care that will be acceptable to both the clinician and the patient.

With its wealth of practical information, *Cross-Cultural Caring* will be particularly useful to those working directly with ethnic patients, such as nurses, social workers, physicians, dentists, and psychologists. It will also provide important information for administrators in health care and social service agencies and will be of interest to those in medical sociology and anthropology.

NANCY WAXLER-MORRISON is an associate professor of social work and sociology at the University of British Columbia.
JOAN M. ANDERSON is a professor of nursing at the University of British Columbia.
ELIZABETH RICHARDSON is a social worker with the Ministry of Social Services and Housing, British Columbia.

Cross-Cultural Caring:
A Handbook for Health
Professionals in Western Canada

Edited by Nancy Waxler-Morrison,
Joan M. Anderson, and
Elizabeth Richardson

University of British Columbia Press
Vancouver 1990

© The University of British Columbia Press 1990
Reprinted 1991
Reprinted 1992
ISBN 0-7748-0343-6

Printed in Canada on acid-free paper ∞

This book has been published
with the help of a grant from
Multiculturalism Canada

Canadian Cataloguing in Publication Data

Main entry under title:
Cross-cultural caring

Includes bibliographical references.
ISBN 0-7748-0343-6

1. Minorities – Medical care – Canada,
Western. 2. Medical anthropology – Canada,
Western. 3. Medical personnel and patient –
Canada, Western. 4. Health attitudes –
Canada, Western – Cross-cultural studies.
I. Waxler-Morrison, Nancy, 1931–   II.
Anderson, Joan Madge, 1940–   III.
Richardson, Elizabeth.
RA563.M56C76 1990   362.1'0425   C89-091578-4

UBC Press
6344 Memorial Rd.
Vancouver, B.C. V6T 1Z2

Contents

Acknowledgments vii
Contributors ix

1 Introduction 3
Nancy Waxler-Morrison

2 The Cambodians and Laotians 11
Elizabeth Richardson

3 The Central Americans 36
Danica Gleave and Arturo S. Manes

4 The Chinese 68
Magdalene C. Lai and Ka-Ming Kevin Yue

5 The Iranians 91
Afsaneh Behjati-Sabet

6 The Japanese 116
Teruko Okabe, Kazuko Takahashi, and Elizabeth Richardson

7 The South Asians 141
Shashi Assanand, Maud Dias, Elizabeth Richardson, and Nancy
Waxler-Morrison

8 The Vietnamese 181
Dai-Kha Dinh, Soma Ganesan, and Nancy Waxler-Morrison

9 The West Indians 214
Joseph H. Glasgow and Eleanor J. Adaskin

Contents

10   Conclusion: Delivering Culturally Sensitive Health Care   245
Joan M. Anderson, Nancy Waxler-Morrison, Elizabeth Richardson,
Carol Herbert, and Maureen Murphy

Appendix: Immigration Regulations and Provision
of Health Services to Immigrants   269
Danica Gleave

Acknowledgments

We are grateful to Glenn Drover and Susan Marshall of the University of British Columbia's School of Social Work for their support and administrative assistance and to Rachel Rousseau, Department of Asian Studies, for her exceptionally competent typing of the manuscript. Thanks, too, to Peter Colenbrander for his skilful editorial work.

We are pleased to acknowledge, with thanks, the generous supporting grants from the Secretary of State and the Vancouver Foundation.

Many members of the immigrant communities as well as many health professionals provided us with invaluable information that could be obtained in no other way. Their names appear at the end of each chapter. Here we wish to thank them for their help and to join with them in the hope that this book will contribute to a form of health care that is both more effective and more acceptable to all Canadians.

Nancy Waxler-Morrison
Joan M. Anderson
Elizabeth Richardson

Contributors

Eleanor J. Adaskin was born and brought up in Manitoba. She is a Clinical Nurse Specialist at the St. Boniface General Hospital in Winnipeg, was educated in Saskatchewan and Washington, and received her Ph.D. in Nursing from the University of Texas at Austin.

Joan M. Anderson is a Professor and National Health Research Scholar in the School of Nursing at UBC. She studied at UBC and McGill universities and received her Ph.D. in Sociology from UBC. She has done research in Canada on immigrant women, including those from Chinese, East Indian, and southern European backgrounds. She was born in Jamaica.

Shashi Assanand was born and raised in Uganda and India. She is a registered social worker at OASIS Immigrant Services Centre in Vancouver and undertakes family and crisis work with members of the South Asian community.

Afsaneh Behjati-Sabet is from Tehran, Iran, where she studied psychology. After coming to Canada she completed an MA in Counselling Psychology at UBC and now works as an employment counsellor at the Surrey-Delta (BC) Immigrant Services Society.

Maud Dias was born in that part of India which later became Pakistan. She is a registered social worker, holds an MSW from Pakistan and now serves as the Volunteer and Programme Co-ordinator for OASIS Immigrant Services Centre in Vancouver.

Dai-Kha Dinh is a family physician in Richmond, BC, who was born in Vinh-yen City in Vietnam and received his MD from the University of Saigon. He has also done further specialty training in France and Quebec.

Soma Ganesan was born and grew up in Vietnam, where he received his MD from the University of Saigon. He is a Clinical Instructor in Psychiatry at UBC and also works at Vancouver General Hospital.

Joseph H. Glasgow is a community mental health worker with the provincial Department of Health in Winnipeg, Manitoba. He was trained as a psychiatric nurse in England. He was born in Trinidad and grew up in Trinidad and England.

Danica Gleave was born in BC and is a graduate of UBC, where she received a BA in anthropology. Most recently she has worked as a research assistant at UBC.

Carol Herbert is Professor and Head of the Department of Family Practice at UBC. She was born and brought up in Vancouver and received her MD and specialty training at UBC.

Magdalene C. Lai recently completed her M.Sc. in Nursing at UBC and has returned to her position as a community health nurse in the Vancouver Health Department's East Unit. She was born in Hong Kong and came to Canada when she was sixteen.

Arturo S. Manes was born in Santiago, Chile, to parents who had migrated there from Germany. He did undergraduate studies in Santiago and received his MD and specialty training at UBC. He is a family physician in Vancouver and has many Latin American patients.

Maureen Murphy, formerly with the UBC School of Nursing and the Vancouver Health Department, is now Director of Public Health Nursing in Ottawa. She was born in Ontario and educated at the University of Western Ontario, where she received her MSN.

Teruko Okabe was born and brought up in Japan, where she studied sociology and received an MA in Educational Psychology in Kyoto. Since coming to live in BC she has become a registered social worker and an instructor at the Centre for Continuing Education at UBC.

Elizabeth Richardson was born and grew up in India, where her Canadian parents lived for many years. She was educated at UBC and at McMaster University from which she received an MA in Sociology, and has taught English in Japan. Currently she works as a social worker for the BC government in North and West Vancouver.

Kazuko Takahashi is a registered nurse, now retired, who was born in BC and received a BSN from UBC. Like many Canadian citizens of

Japanese descent she lived in government relocation camps during the Second World War.

Nancy Waxler-Morrison is an Associate Professor in the School of Social Work and the Department of Anthropology and Sociology at UBC. She was born and received her early education in Illinois and received a Ph.D. in sociology from Harvard. She has done research in the medical sociology field in Sri Lanka.

Ka-Ming Kevin Yue is a family physician who practises in Vancouver. He was born in Canton, China, grew up in Hong Kong, and received his MD and family physician specialty training at UBC.

Cross-Cultural Caring

CHAPTER ONE

Introduction

Nancy Waxler-Morrison

Mrs. L., a social worker at the public health department in a small town in western Canada received a call from Dr. N., a local GP who said, "I've just examined a two-year-old child from one of those Vietnamese families living out north of town. He's got bruises all over his back and I think you had better make a home visit because it looks like a case of child abuse to me. We'll probably have to report it." Mrs. L. discovered that the family lived in a trailer park full of Vietnamese refugees. The mother worked as a cleaner in the local hospital; the father was unemployed and stayed at home with their four young children. The two-year-old had had a severe cold and trouble breathing, which led the parents to take him to the doctor. When Mrs. L. looked at the child she too saw bruise marks down his back. The child's mother looked somewhat embarrassed as she explained that they were short of money so didn't take him to the doctor right away but instead tried a treatment everyone used in Vietnam—"spooning." A silver spoon was pressed firmly up and down the child's back as a way to remove the illness. That's where the bruises had come from. They had done this for about five days but since it hadn't seemed to work they had finally taken the child to the doctor.

PURPOSE OF THIS BOOK

The potential "problem" in the Vietnamese family described above arises not simply from the use of a traditional healing practice that many Western practitioners would think useless or even harmful because it delays good treatment. It also arises from the Western practitioner's assumptions that parents may harm children and that the government may or should intervene. Thus both Vietnamese parents and Western-trained GP's have ways of understanding and treating illness that derive from the culture in which they live. These "cultures of medicine" are often incongruent. It is the avoidance of this "clash of cultures" and the resulting dissatisfaction and poor health care that we address in this book. For health professionals we hope to provide knowledge about the social background, beliefs, and practices of particular cultural groups in order to ease patient management. For members of various immigrant groups in western Canada we hope to provide guidelines that will ensure that their expectations, needs, and interests are attended to when they need health care.

How are ethnic and cultural factors associated with health and health care? First, some diseases are associated with ethnic group membership. These diseases may be genetically linked, prevalent in the home country because it is poor and poorly served by preventive medicine, or linked to diet or other cultural practices. Because these culturally linked diseases are often unusual and not a central part of Western medical training, knowledge of them is obviously useful to professionals. Second, ethnic membership often means family structure, religion, medical beliefs, and practices which are incongruent with Western society or its health beliefs, thus leading to unfulfilled expectations and dissatisfied doctors and patients. Third, these incongruencies often result in ineffective health care, to patient non-compliance, from the point of view of the practitioner, and to continued illness, alienation, and feelings of being discriminated against, from the point of view of the ethnic patient.

This handbook will provide the health practitioner with basic information about some immigrant groups in western Canada. Major attention will be paid to the social contexts in which ethnic patients live: why they came to Canada, where and how they live, what sort of family situation is common, who provides support, who makes decisions, what medical practices and beliefs they have brought from their home countries, and what problems they experience in obtaining health care in Canada. Such concrete information about immigrant groups may aid professionals in providing more culturally sensitive health care.

PERSPECTIVE

It is not only the recent immigrants in the West who have distinctive cultures, including medicine. They do indeed bring with them beliefs about what causes symptoms—everything from the "evil eye" to "too much bile gone to the head" to "germs"—and about suitable treatments, ranging from talismans to aspirin to coriander tea. But Western-trained health professionals—(usually) white Canadian doctors and nurses who provide health care—also have a distinctive "culture of health," often taken for granted and thus unrecognized. Western health professionals often attribute disease to individual behaviour, such as exposing oneself to germs or eating improperly, and believe that the individual is thus largely responsible for getting well. Getting well usually means co-operation with technical procedures applied to the body such as medicines and surgery.

Health care is a social process in which each party—the professional and the patient—brings a set of beliefs, expectations, and practices to the encounter. Their common task is to negotiate an understanding of the problem, or diagnosis, and decide what to do about it. Health practitioners usually do not think of their day-to-day work in these terms. Instead, they use phrases like "taking the history," "physical examination," or "management" to describe medical work as a technical task to which they apply their expertise and training. It is easy to think in these terms when the health practitioner and the patient share very basic assumptions about illness and treatment. If both are members of the Canadian cultural majority, it is likely that they will share a culture of medicine in which the patient and the practitioner both believe that bacteria and viruses, for example, cause disease; that the patient should provide concise and relevant information about his or her symptoms to the doctor; and that the patient should follow the technical recommendations of the health professional if the illness is to be cured. Negotiations between a doctor and a patient who share a common culture are often smooth and satisfying to both parties.

When the same health professional treats a patient who has a different culture of medicine such negotiations are often ineffective and unsatisfactory to both. This is often the case in western Canada when the patient belongs to an immigrant cultural group. The professional's culture—in which medical care is largely a technical task requiring the individual co-operation of the patient—clashes with the patient's culture of medicine. For example, in some non-Western cultures the patient is expected to wait passively for the doctor's diagnosis since "the doctor should know" what the problem is. Western-style taking of histories is not part of the patient's experience. Or, in some cultures, whether or not a sick family member takes the prescribed medicine is not his or her decision but the prerogative of the family head, who is often the grandfather or grandmother. Instructions or recommendations by health professional to patient, stemming from our Western concern with individual responsibility, are thus ineffective.

Both the Western culture of medicine of most Canadian health professionals and an immigrant or minority patient's culture of medicine are legitimate perspectives. The Western biomedical system does not have a monopoly of wisdom on how a sick person should behave, the kinds of recommendations a health professional should make, or even on understanding the etiology of disease. Thus, it is unrealistic and unhelpful to ignore cultural differences and to hope that Western medical practices will always work smoothly or that the ethnic patient will simply adapt to them. Instead, if the professional is alert to his or her own culture of medicine and has some understanding of other cultures it is more likely that a mutually satisfactory agreement can be made about how to deal with the problem. The professional is more likely to achieve "compliance" or effective treatment and the patient more likely to recover and feel satisfied.

Cross-Cultural Caring provides a basic introduction to the social background and culture of a number of immigrant groups in western Canada. Comprehensive knowledge about every ethnic group is impossible and unnecessary, so we have not attempted to furnish it. In fact, each member of a cultural group will be somewhat different from his or her own cultural counterparts. What we have done is to alert health practitioners and other professionals to some of the important cultural characteristics. These can be explored in more detail with an individual patient or family. In the last chapter, we suggest culturally sensitive ways of obtaining important information from patients and their families, of negotiating common understanding, and of agreeing upon care plans that are consistent with the cultures of both health practitioner and patient.

COMMON PROBLEMS OF ETHNIC AND CULTURAL MINORITIES IN WESTERN CANADA

Although each cultural minority group has a distinct history, social situation, and set of beliefs, they have some experiences and problems in common. These are often reflected in their use of health services, their experiences with health professionals, and their common illnesses. Some of these problems appear over and over again in the chapters that follow.

Many of the cultural minorities described are relatively recent migrants to Canada. The disruption of life associated with migration affects many people from different cultures in similar ways. Much has been lost: family ties, familiar language, community support, the comfort that comes from the general predictability of life. Some migrants, too, have not lost the familiar life by choice; some *have* come to Canada to better their lives but others have come as refugees. Recent migrants have lost a great deal and need strength to reintegrate and begin again.

Migration also requires adaptation to a new society. Many migrants must learn a new language, find new supports, change how they eat, live, and relate to their own children. They must also learn new jobs, and create new visions of the future. Dealing with adaptation, like dealing with loss, takes time and energy.

Three problems are felt by almost all cultural groups, particularly early in their stay in Canada. The first is lack of English. Many are eager to learn and do so quickly, but lack of English makes all health service encounters frustrating and often unrewarding for everyone, and the help available for the problem in no way meets the need. Second is lack of money. Some immigrants have or can bring funds to cover living expenses; others rely on relatives in Canada. The majority often live at a basic subsistence level and find it difficult, for example, to buy medicine and to pay for bus fares to the hospital. The third problem is the health, social service, and immigration bureaucracy which, for many, is difficult to understand and to utilize. Many people spend scarce time and money going from one office to another to obtain clarification of status and medical insurance. (The appendix includes a brief description of Department of Immigration and Employment procedures, classifications, and policies about health care, as of 1989.)

Just as there are common problems for most new immigrants, there are issues specific to members of particular immigrant families. Especially crucial for many immigrant women is learning to balance housework and a paid job without the support of the family network that they once had at home. Also, immigrant women are often the last to learn the new language, resulting in social isolation and an inability to use the help that is available. Men, too, often experience loss of status and self-esteem since jobs for which they were trained in their home countries are often closed to them in Canada; doctors may work as hospital orderlies and teachers as store clerks. Family relationships often change. Children usually learn English sooner and therefore become intermediaries between parents and the outside world, and therefore displace the father from his former role. Moreover, children generally adopt Western dress, behaviour, and aspirations which are often believed by their parents to be bad, immoral, or disrespectful. The resultant personal and

family stresses may lead to both physical and mental health problems.

Members of these cultural minority groups frequently experience
problems with hospitals and health professionals that represent, in
microcosm, the general difficulties they have in the new society.
They feel frustrated and insecure because few health professionals
can communicate in the family's language and translators are not
readily available. Even if someone in the family can speak English,
the family's lack of understanding about how the health system
works and the health professional's unawareness of the need for
explanation may mean wasted time and energy which working family members can ill afford. Many members of cultural minorities feel
that health professionals do not understand them but instead simply assume that they feel and believe just as other Canadians do.
Some experience their contact with health professionals as "stereotyping"; for example, behaving towards them as if "all East Indians
are the same." Some report encounters in hospitals and clinics in
terms of discrimination, prejudice, or racism.

Health professionals' problems in working with cultural minority
groups include patients not following instructions, and medicines
not being taken or being given to another family member with a
different disease. Families may not abide by hospital policies and
instead may visit in large numbers, bringing small children and
forbidden food. Parents may not dress their small children properly
or provide nutritious food or may send sick children to school.
Appointments may be missed, advice not followed. Health professionals often see real problems in providing what they believe to be
good care to many immigrant and minority group patients.

Some of these "problems," as seen by minority group members or
by health professionals, are linked to incongruent cultures of health.
Each party often has distinctly different understandings of illness,
beliefs about appropriate behaviour for doctors and sick people, and
ideas about proper treatment. Compounding this is the fact that
health professionals, mostly members of the majority culture, are
very powerful relative to patients. Professionals have or are believed
to have, the expertise, that the patient lacks; this expertise is the
reason for seeking professional care in the first place. Professionals
have even greater power and control when they belong to the majority culture and treat members of the minority. In this case it is
extremely difficult for the patient or his family to ask questions, seek
a second opinion, or disagree with the proposed treatment. Differences in relative power between professional and patient simply

compound the problems ethnic minority members and health professionals have in collaborating with each other.

IMMIGRANT GROUPS DESCRIBED

We have not tried to describe all immigrant groups in western Canada, nor to focus on the largest groups or even the most recent arrivals. Instead, we have selected the people who report that they have the most problems in obtaining satisfactory health care, and/or those cultural groups believed by health professionals to be the most difficult to work with. In short, we describe people who have "problems" with health care.

Problems in any segment of the Canadian population can certainly be found and consequently our selection is somewhat arbitrary and subjective. It is not implied that other cultural groups have no problems in obtaining satisfactory health care. However, the groups we have chosen provide useful insights into the variety of these problems and the solutions to them.

While other cultural groups in Canada—notably Native Indians and Inuit—are sometimes dissatisfied with mainstream health care, they are not discussed in this book for the obvious reason that they are not immigrants. Also not covered is the predominant Anglo-Canadian group which has its own "culture of health." All of these groups deserve attention in further publications.

The immigrant groups we describe represent minority cultures: South Asians, Japanese, Chinese, Vietnamese, Iranians, Central Americans, Cambodians, Laotians, and West Indians. We describe them in terms of their country or area of origin. Many members of these groups in Canada are Canadian citizens or will become so.

What is meant by "cultural minority?" These are distinctive and identifiable subgroups in the Canadian population which see themselves as having origins, beliefs, and values in common. In a word, they share a distinctive culture. This is a "minority" culture because it contrasts with the culture of the largest and most powerful subgroup of the population, the white, European culture. Underlying this contrast is a distinction in economic and political power as well. Although cultural minority groups *do* hold distinct beliefs about "right" behaviour and values, and about appropriate responses to misbehaviour, they are often less well-off and have less political power than the majority. Therefore, minority culture often implies both distinctive cultural beliefs and less powerful social positions. Both characteristics are reflected in the problems these sub-groups and health professionals have in devising mutually satisfactory health care.

When describing a cultural group there is always the danger of stereotyping, of implying all group members are the same. Yet if one takes the opposite position—that the group is only a collection of unique individuals—one would deny the reality of a common culture that is taught to each individual to ensure that the society survives. In practice, we know that East Indians generally believe that imbalance in the body humours causes illness and that a diet of hot and cool foods may relieve the symptoms. Yet we also know that some East Indians who come to Canada are Westernized and do not really believe in the idea of imbalance. Thus to recognize diversity and avoid stereotyping we attempt to point out important variations within each cultural minority group. Thereafter it is up to the health professional to investigate carefully each patient's circumstances so as to understand that individual's "culture of health."

HOW THIS BOOK WAS WRITTEN

We have asked members of cultural minority groups to speak for themselves, through the authors of each chapter. In most cases, authors are members of the same cultural group, and are health or social service professionals with day-to-day experience with patients and families from that group. They have drawn upon their own experiences as well as their cultural knowledge. The validity of each chapter was checked by other members of the cultural group. Sometimes a person has a blind spot about his own culture. For that reason we asked professionals who work with, but do not belong to, that cultural group to read and comment on the work. Thus each chapter is the work of one or more people who were helped by a number of others. All the contributors are listed at the end of each chapter.

CHAPTER TWO

The Cambodians and Laotians
Elizabeth Richardson

Although Cambodian and Laotian immigrants in Canada are discussed jointly in this chapter, they are linguistically and culturally distinct from each other and form socially separate communities. They nevertheless share certain historical and cultural features including the fact that the overwhelming majority in both communities are refugees.

Most Cambodians and Laotians in Canada differ from other immigrants in that the decision to leave their home countries was largely forced on them by political and economic upheavals beyond their control. In this sense, migration was neither voluntary nor planned. Refugees also have in common the general fact that their departures were hurried and dramatic, and that during their flight many suffered extreme physical and emotional hardship, starvation, disease, loss of and separation from family and friends, financial loss, and so on. In most cases, escape from their homelands was followed by long periods of uncertainty in crowded refugee camps, where insanitary conditions and insufficient food and medical supplies were not uncommon. In the meantime they had to wait to be accepted by whichever host country would take them. Acceptance by Canadian immigration authorities and arrival in Canada, while solving many problems, added others. These were culture shock, language difficulties, financial worries, and unemployment or underemployment. At the same time as these refugees are attempting to settle in and adjust to Canada, they must also come to terms with the permanent loss of their homes. Many dream of returning home some day and this can make adaptation in Canada even more difficult.

Cambodia and Laos are neighbouring countries in Southeast Asia, and have some common historical and cultural characteristics. Both experienced the early influence of Indian culture, and they share the

Theravada Buddhist religious tradition. They both formed part of French Indochina and remained French colonies until independence in 1953. As a consequence of the colonial era, both countries inherited a legacy of French language and culture. During the colonial period, large numbers of Chinese migrated to Indochina as traders and merchants, and eventually gained control of the rice and sugar industries. They remained a distinct ethnic minority in both countries and were generally resented by the majority because of their dominant economic position. Also during the colonial period, Vietnamese were brought in by the French to man much of the government bureaucracy. This imposition of foreign authority strengthened the historical antipathy of Cambodians and Laotians towards the Vietnamese as a result of earlier conflicts.

CAMBODIA

Cambodia, or the People's Republic of Kampuchea as it is now known officially, is a tropical country situated in the southwestern part of the Indochinese peninsula, and is bounded by Thailand, Laos, and Vietnam, with a southwest seacoast on the Gulf of Siam. The climate is hot and humid with monsoon rains in the summer.

Prior to the communist takeover of the country in 1975, the economy was based on agriculture with exports of rice, corn, rubber, and textiles. Since then, the country has been in a state of economic collapse.

The population comprises three main ethnic groups, the largest being the Khmer representing roughly 85 per cent, with Vietnamese and Chinese each making up about 5 per cent of the total. Traditionally, the majority of ethnic Khmer were farmers working primarily in rice cultivation, while the Chinese minority were urban dwellers involved in business enterprises.

History and Reasons for Migration

Following independence from France, Cambodia became a constitutional monarchy under Prince Norodom Sihanouk. In 1970, Sihanouk was overthrown by a military coup and the new pro-American, anti-communist regime was headed by General Lon Nol. Fighting ensued between government forces and the communist Khmer Rouge, and ended in victory for the Khmer Rouge in 1975, with Pol Pot leading the new government.

The situation in Cambodia in the three years which followed has been described as genocide. Upon seizing power in 1975, the Pol Pot regime embarked on a policy of de-urbanizing the country. Cities were forcibly evacuated and urban dwellers were expected to join the peasantry in agricultural production. Buddhism was disestablished as the state religion and other religions were also suppressed. Markets and money were abolished. Educational institutions and medical care were disrupted. Those who were educated, had exposure to Western culture, were associated with the previous regime, or who resisted the new one were executed or severely persecuted. Thousands of others died as a result of starvation and disease. Food was inadequate and medical care was minimal. To attempt escape was a crime punishable by death. Nonetheless many did manage to flee to Thailand or Vietnam, some of them walking for as long as two months, day and night, and suffering from malnutrition and disease en route (Garry 1980; Kiljunun 1984).

In 1979, Vietnam invaded Cambodia and set up a puppet government. By 1989 negotiations were under way to withdraw Vietnamese forces and to set up a new Cambodian government.

Cambodian immigration to Canada essentially dates from 1979. Between 1975 and 1979, it was extremely difficult to get out of the country, but following the overthrow of the Pol Pot regime, there was greater freedom of movement and opportunity to escape. The number of immigrants to Canada peaked in 1980 at approximately 3000. Since then, the yearly average has been about 1500.

LAOS

Laos is a small, land-locked country comprising densely wooded mountains and fertile river valleys with a tropical monsoon climate. Laos shares borders with Vietnam, Cambodia, Thailand, and in the north, with Burma and China. The country has been traditionally agricultural, producing rice, corn, tobacco, coffee, and cotton, and the majority of the population are farmers living in lowland river valleys in small rural villages.

About 50 per cent of the population are ethnic Lao who are farmers or educated urban lowlanders. Of the several minority groups, one of the largest is the Hmong, a generally illiterate mountain people who have retained a distinctive language and cultural tradition. The Chinese also constitute a minority and were traditionally city dwellers involved in business enterprises (Royle 1980).

History and Reasons for Migration

Following independence in 1953, fighting broke out between the

Royal Lao government and the pro-communist Pathet Lao. A period of almost continuous warfare ensued, with the French and later the United States supporting the Royal Lao government, and the Vietnamese communists backing the Pathet Lao. During this period of civil war, families were uprooted and driven from their homes. In 1975, following communist victories in Cambodia and Vietnam, the Pathet Lao took control of the country. Since that time, large numbers of refugees have fled to camps in Thailand. Economic collapse caused by drought and bad harvests, along with the new government's policy of reprisals against those who supported the former regime, largely contributed to the exodus. Initially, refugees were from the upper and middle classes—professionals, students, merchants, and administrative and technical employees of the former regime. As the economic situation deteriorated and resistance to the new government increased, Laotians from rural areas joined the exodus. Another major refugee group from Laos was the Hmong, the rural hill people mentioned above, most of whom found asylum in the United States. Few came to Canada (Asia Survey 1973–88).

In order to escape from Laos, refugees had to cross the Mekong River to get to Thailand. This was done by swimming or by paying for transportation in boats, and sometimes those who were caught were shot. As with the Cambodians, most of the Laotian refugees underwent extreme physical and emotional hardship while escaping and during their ensuing lengthy internment in Thai camps. Immigration to Canada basically dates from 1979 when the largest number of refugees, close to 4000, was accepted. In recent years, the average number has been about 700.

Socio-Economic Factors

There is considerable diversity in the socio-economic backgrounds of the refugees from Cambodia and Laos. Some are well-educated and formerly lived in urban areas in their home countries, while others have rural origins, little formal schooling, and limited prior exposure to Western technology. Clearly, the experiences of these refugees in adjusting to Canadian society, including the health care system, will differ widely.

As mentioned above, many urban, educated, middle-class Cambodians were either executed by the Pol Pot regime or fled when it assumed power. Consequently by 1979 when Cambodian migration to Canada began in earnest, the majority of the refugees were drawn from the countryside. Most were farmers and labourers and many have not completed high school. The Cambodian population in Canada is mostly young, and made up of family groups although there are many single people. The elderly comprise only a very small percentage. The vast majority were sponsored by the federal government, unlike many Laotians who were sponsored privately by church groups, for example. The majority of Cambodians in BC live in the Lower Mainland, and there is a large population in Edmonton, Alberta.

In general, knowledge of English in Canada's Cambodian community is very poor and as a result jobs tend to be unskilled and poorly paid. Many families are forced to supplement part-time or marginal incomes with financial assistance from the government. It has been noted that Cambodians "have been the least well served by public and private attempts at refugee assistance and have had to carry on primarily on their own. This has led to difficulties in finding employment, underuse of social and health services, social isolation, and a lack of public and government awareness of Khmer [Cambodian] problems and concerns" (Indra 1985:456).

Downward occupational mobility has been common among Laotian refugees due to poor mastery of English and an inability to find employment in occupations for which they were previously trained. Furthermore, they lack time and money for retraining as their immediate priority is to support their families. The overwhelming majority do not have the same type of employment as they had in their home country. Former teachers, army officers, administrative personnel, and technicians may be found employed as farmworkers, factory workers, and janitorial staff, positions they would never have considered at home because of their education, training, and social status.

The Laotian community in Canada is made up primarily of young families; there are very few elderly. The majority were sponsored privately and the community tends to be widely scattered because people settled near their sponsors.

A significant number of both Cambodians and Laotians are ethnic Chinese who, as a minority group, have retained their own language, religion, and cultural traditions. Once in Canada, they tend to identify more with other Chinese Canadians than with their former fellow nationals, and gravitate towards the Chinese community.

Finances and employment are extremely high priority issues for most Cambodians and Laotians in Canada. Generally, their savings were used up during their escape and in the refugee camps, and many feel obliged to send money to assist relatives still in Southeast Asia. Underemployment can lead to frustration, humiliation, and depression, and is especially difficult for members of these cultures because class and status distinctions are taken very seriously. Many refugees have had periods of unemployment due to lay-offs from marginal jobs and this experience can cause feelings of shame and incompetence, and can affect familial and social relationships.

Special Problems in Canada

Cambodian immigrants to Canada cannot sponsor the immigration of family members from Cambodia as the present Vietnamese-backed regime is not officially recognized by the Canadian government. Only family members who have managed to escape to refugee camps outside the country can be sponsored. Consequently, many Cambodians have no relatives in Canada and commonly experience feelings of isolation and homesickness.

EXPERIENCE WITH CANADIANS

Cambodians and Laotians from rural areas are used to friendly, relaxed relationships with neighbours. Doors and windows are left open and neighbours' voices carry easily from one house to the next. These immigrants frequently experience a major difference in Canadian neighbourhood life, finding that Canadians are quiet and keep to themselves. Many feel lonely and isolated as a result.

LANGUAGE

As noted previously, French was the language of government, business, and education during the colonial period in Indochina, and as a result, many Cambodians and Laotians who are over the age of forty speak or are familiar with French. However, few had experience of English before coming to Canada, although those with some French have an easier time learning the language.

The predominant language in Laos is Lao, a member of the Sino-Tibetan family of languages. In Cambodia, the predominant language is Khmer. The Chinese established their own schools where possible in Cambodia and Laos, and have retained their own language.

RELIGION

Cambodian and Laotian cultures are similar largely because of the influence of Theravada Buddhism, one of the main streams of Buddhist thought, which is adhered to by 90 per cent of the population of both countries. The majority of the Chinese follow the beliefs of Mahayana Buddhism, the Chinese school of Buddhism which is also practised in Vietnam. A notion central to Buddhism is that desire for pleasure and possessions causes suffering which, however, can be avoided through non-attachment to things. In other words, man can avoid undue pain and suffering through moderation in all aspects of behaviour, including the expression of strong emotions. Another basic and interconnected belief is reincarnation and the theory of karma; that is, that one's present life is the consequence of one's deeds in a previous one. Through correct and meritorious behaviour, man can improve the condition of his next life. Buddhism tends to be family-centred and rituals are frequently practised in the home.

Before the advent of Buddhism in Cambodia and Laos, there existed an animistic cult marked by the worship of spirits which lived in people and in nature. In Laos, for example, there was an ancient belief in thirty-two spirits which inhabited the human body. At the time of death, these spirits were believed to separate and then combine with others to be reborn in a new body. However, the spirits of those who died in childbirth, accidents, or other violent causes were considered evil and were prevented from being reborn. More precisely, these spirits were doomed to roam the earth, tormenting the lives of others by, for example, causing physical or mental illness (Oberg and Deinard 1984). Such animistic beliefs continue to be held in varying degrees, particularly by those from rural backgrounds, and co-exist with Buddhist tenets.

At present, there is no temple for Cambodian and Laotian Buddhists in BC; the closest is in Seattle. However, the Laotian community in the Lower Mainland is attempting to raise funds to bring in and support a Buddhist monk to serve its religious needs.

FAMILY STRUCTURE

Traditionally in Cambodian and Laotian society, the family is the key social and economic unit. The extended family forms a network of support and assistance, both financial and emotional. The role of women is subordinate, although relative to some other parts of Asia, their status is quite high. They are responsible for child-rearing, for performing most household duties, and commonly, for managing family finances. They are expected by men to be virtuous, gentle, modest, and obedient. The husband as head of the household has authority, and is the decisionmaker and breadwinner. Typically, in

Southeast Asia, women are not employed outside the home, although in recent years in Cambodia, many were forced to support families when husbands and male relatives died in the war or were conscripted for military service.

In Cambodia, the Pol Pot regime, fearing conspiracy, discouraged close family relationships. Many policies were aimed at weakening traditionally strong family ties: family members were encouraged to spy and report on one another; children were taught to distrust parents. These experiences may continue to affect family relationships and attitudes in Canada.

In urban areas of Cambodia and Laos, a household usually consists of a married couple and their unmarried children. In rural areas of Laos, households tend to be extended, while in Cambodia they are nuclear. In Canada, where low income levels are common, households are often shared with other adult relatives so that several income earners live together, thereby allowing all to enjoy a higher standard of living.

Family problems are considered personal and private. Solutions are sought within the family, or sometimes with the assistance of close friends. However, in most cases, the doors are firmly closed to involvement by outsiders, including professionals.

MARRIAGE

In Laos and Cambodia, marriages are typically arranged in the sense that the parents of both partners are closely involved. However, the wishes of the young couple are taken into consideration. The man's family is generally interested in the girl's character, social reputation, and ability to perform household tasks. The concerns of the girl's family include her prospective husband's character, family background, and social status. Dating is rare and courting takes the form of group activities, such as parties, and is seen as leading to marriage. Premarital chastity for women is highly valued and an unwed girl who becomes pregnant brings shame to her family. In rural areas she may be considered an evil person who will attract bad fortune. Divorce is rare and disapproved of strongly.

Following a wedding in Cambodia, the young couple lives with or near the bride's family. In Laos, the couple generally starts married life with the bride's family, sometimes moving later to the husband's family home, or out on their own. Young married couples in Canada usually live independently from the outset.

CHILD-REARING

Children are taught to respect and obey parents and other adults. There is a hierarchical order among siblings whereby the younger ones are expected to defer to and respect the older ones, who in turn, are often required to care for their juniors. This is particularly true in the case of the eldest male child, who in his teenage years has almost parental authority and responsibility for his younger siblings.

Infants are seldom allowed to cry, are carried more, and tend to walk later than Canadian children. Generally breast-feeding continues longer and toilet-training, which is learned through observation rather than deliberate conditioning, comes later. For the most part, there is a more relaxed attitude towards the stages of childhood. From infancy, children take their place at social events, ceremonies, and so on. They are not excluded from family activities because of age and would, for example, be allowed to stay up late when parents entertain.

Discipline is rarely physical, especially for young children. Instead, it generally takes the form of persistent verbal admonition. Children are expected to learn correct behaviour by observing and imitating adults. However, they are generally more strictly controlled than Canadian children. For example, open disagreement with parents would be unusual.

Cambodian and Laotian cultures are very protective of girls, who tend to be brought up more strictly than boys because their reputations must be beyond reproach if a suitable marriage partner is to be found. They are taught a helping role within the family, are given a greater share of household tasks, and are, traditionally, not expected to achieve the same level of education as the boys. In Canada, many parents place a high priority on education for children of both sexes as it is seen as the key to upward mobility.

THE ELDERLY

The elderly have great authority and receive considerable respect in traditional Laotian and Cambodian societies, particularly the men, who are called on to advise and to make important decisions for family members.

Typically, elderly parents live with their families, never alone, and adult children feel a strong responsibility to care for them. In these extended families grandparents give practical help with household tasks and often with the care of grandchildren.

SPECIAL PROBLEMS RESULTING FROM MIGRATION

Refugees from Cambodia and Laos have experienced the instability of years of warfare and of long periods of dislocation in refugee camps, as well as loss of and separation from family members. All of this has placed a tremendous strain on the traditional structure of the family. To these factors are added the severe stresses of adjusting to life in Canada which further contribute to the potential breakdown of traditional family patterns, and to family problems and conflict.

School children are caught between two cultures. On the one hand are the traditional values of their parents, and on the other is the pressure to conform to peer values and behaviour. They may expect more freedom and be less willing to defer to the authority of parents and older relatives. They may experience confusion, loneliness, and alienation in a school environment which differs so greatly from that in their home countries. The role of the teacher, which at home is highly authoritarian, is here very much more relaxed and familiar. Behavioural expectations are different; for example, children may be extremely embarrassed at having to undress in school locker rooms and may consequently avoid activities such as gym and swimming.

Parenting becomes much more difficult in a new culture. Children usually adapt more readily and acquire the English language more quickly than their parents. This frequently leads to a role reversal where parents rely on children for information and interpretation, a situation which can ultimately lead to the undermining of parental dignity and authority. Parents of teenagers, especially girls, may be concerned about the freedom adolescents enjoy in Canada relative to the home countries, where dating is not acceptable and where male and female teenagers generally do not spend time together alone. In short, many parents feel that in Canadian society, children and adolescents are accorded rights and privileges by schools, social services, and so on, which threaten their traditional authority and control.

Many Cambodian families with teenagers have an especially difficult time in Canada. As has been noted above, during the Pol Pot regime, children were frequently indoctrinated to distrust parents as possible enemies of the state, and were taught to protect the revolution by informing on their families. Many were separated from their parents and lived for long periods in collective work camps or training schools. Such children who are now teenagers in Canada tend to have family and school problems. They may have difficulty in coping with other students and with school work, and sometimes drop out.

Whereas previously the large majority of Cambodian and Laotian women did not work outside the home, many are forced to do so out of economic necessity in Canada. This change can upset the traditional family balance in which the woman was financially dependent on her husband, and can undermine the self-esteem of men, whose traditional role was that of family breadwinner.

Although the elderly do not form a large proportion of the Cambodian and Laotian communities in Canada, a common problem for those who are here is loneliness and isolation. An elderly Cambodian woman recalls: "When I stayed in the refugee camps, I had many friends. I was very poor and didn't have enough food, but I had friends." In an unfamiliar culture, with minimal language skills, the elderly are likely to experience a loss of traditional status and authority and to feel helpless and dependent on their adult children.

CULTURAL VALUES AND BEHAVIOUR

According to the Laotian naming system, as in Canada, the personal name comes first, followed by the family name. Traditionally the family name is not very important and people are generally addressed and referred to by their personal names. When a Laotian woman marries, she takes her husband's family name. Most Laotian family names are polysyllabic, for example, Koulavongsa or Sysavoth.

In Cambodia, unlike Canada, the family name comes first, followed by the given name. As in Laos, given names are used more frequently than family names. So for example, if a man's family name is Vong and his given name is Sararith, he will be addressed as Mr. Vong Sararith or more commonly, Mr. Sararith. Similarly, if his wife's personal name is Maly, she will be called Mrs. Maly or Mrs. Vong Maly. At the time of marriage, a Cambodian woman takes her husband's family name. A child is often given a nickname shortly after birth, a custom originally intended to confuse the evil spirits which might want to cause harm.

In Southeast Asia, time is generally more elastic than it is in Canada; the pace of life is more relaxed and for the most part punctuality is considered unimportant. However, people adjust quickly to Canadian expectations and keeping appointment times is usually a problem only for some newcomers.

The traditional greeting involves pressing the palms of one's hands together at chest level accompanied by a slight bow. This gesture is also used to express thanks. While some Cambodian and Laotian men have adopted the Western custom of shaking hands, women may not feel comfortable with this practice. Traditionally, the head of the family is greeted first.

Hospitality is a strong tradition in Cambodian and Laotian cultures. The concept of the "Dutch treat" is foreign, and the host is expected to pay for his guests, for example at a restaurant. Casual visits do not require an invitation and there is much entertaining of family and friends at home.

Cambodians and Laotians may initially respond to invitations by refusing so as not to appear over-eager or impolite. Typically, the offer or invitation is then made several times, after which it is considered appropriate to accept.

Gift-giving is less common than among Canadians and is usually not associated with special occasions, except in the case of weddings. Acceptance by a woman of a man's gift signifies encouragement of romantic intentions and may not be considered entirely proper. People may be reluctant to accept favours where they feel unable to reciprocate. Occasionally, thanks may be expressed by giving an extravagant gift.

Physical expressions of affection between members of the opposite sex, including married couples, are considered improper when performed in public or even in front of friends. Body parts are seen to exist in a hierarchy, the most supreme and respected part being the head, with other parts diminishing in importance towards the feet. Touching the head or shoulder of another person in casual contact, particularly if he or she is older, is viewed as extremely disrespectful. When communicating, the avoidance of eye contact is an expression of respect.

For some recent immigrants from rural backgrounds and with little experience of telephones, a telephone conversation may lack the reality of a face-to-face encounter and information received in this manner may not be taken seriously.

In accordance with Buddhist beliefs, the traditional attitude towards life stresses harmony and interdependence; direct confrontation is avoided and the expression of anger or displeasure is considered rude. Conflicts and disagreements are approached indirectly, and a person may simply withdraw when giving offense appears unavoidable. Thus an overt "yes" does not always signify true agreement, but may simply indicate a desire to maintain politeness and harmony. For example, if someone does not wish to see a health professional, he or she may agree to an appointment and then fail to keep it. Similarly, a smile does not necessarily express approval, pleasure, or acceptance; it may only be intended to prevent social discomfort or to conceal anger, embarrrassment, or grief.

In Canada, Cambodians and Laotians wear Western-style clothing, and remove their shoes when entering a home. Some Cambodians and Laotians dislike using second-hand articles, especially clothing. This attitude may stem from fears that the previous owner died, or was a carrier of a communicable disease or general bad luck which might then transfer to the new owner. Hospital gowns, however, are accepted as they are also used in home countries.

Traditionally, in Cambodia and Laos, people sleep on low beds made of wood or bamboo, or on floor mats. In Canada, Western-style beds are used.

Laotians traditionally celebrate a special custom called baci (pronounced "bassi") whereby individuals receive blessings and wishes of good health and prosperity. During the ceremony, cotton strings are tied around the wrists of the persons being honoured and are subsequently worn for three days. Baci is celebrated on many occasions, such as the birth of a baby, marriage, recovery from illness, graduation from high school or university, or to mark any other happy event. It continues to be practised by Laotians living in Canada.

RECREATION AND LEISURE

In Cambodia and Laos sports, especially soccer, are a popular pastime and recreation is generally family-centred. In Canada, families from these countries tend not to spend money on entertainment such as movies, restaurants, or the theatre, but rather enjoy their free time at home or visiting friends and relatives.

FESTIVALS AND HOLIDAYS

Pimay, the Laotian New Year, is the only traditional holiday that continues to be practised by Laotians living in Canada. According to the Buddhist calendar, it falls in early to mid-April and marks the end of Laos's dry season and a return to growth and prosperity. In Canada, it is celebrated by the ceremony of baci, followed by a party with food and dancing.

Cambodians in Canada observe several religious celebrations during the year, with a Buddhist monk officiating when possible. As in the Laotian tradition, the New Year is determined by the Buddhist calendar and is celebrated in April, when the community gathers together for a party.

HEALTH CARE SYSTEMS IN CAMBODIA AND LAOS

There are no medical insurance systems in Cambodia and Laos, and patients are required to pay cash for treatment. Hospitals exist only in major urban centres, and rural areas have few health services, including dental care. People from these areas rarely travel to the cities for treatment because of the expense involved. In most medical centres and offices, patients must wait their turn to see a doctor or nurse as there is no appointment system.

PREVALENT DISEASES

Major health problems in Cambodia and Laos include tuberculosis, malaria, trachoma, diptheria, typhoid, amoebic dysentery, hepatitis, intestinal parasites, malnutrition, beriberi, and kwashiorkor. Moreover, leprosy sometimes occurs in outlying rural areas. Infant mortality rates are high and life expectancy in Cambodia for the period 1980–81 was 44 for males and 46.9 for females; in Laos, it was 39.1 and 41.8 respectively.

Many Cambodians and Laotians arriving at refugee camps in Thailand are ill, and commonly suffer from malnutrition, anaemia, malaria, parasites, and respiratory problems. The often insanitary conditions in the crowded camps, combined with insufficient medical attention, make recovery difficult.

Diseases which have been found in refugees new to Canada include tuberculosis, intestinal parasites, anaemia, hepatitis B, and dental caries. In a study of the health status of Indo-Chinese refugees, recently arrived Cambodians were found to be in poorer health than other groups, probably because of the extreme deprivation they had suffered during the past decade, including lack of food, shelter, and medical care (Catanzaro and Moser 1982). Lactose intolerance, that is, inability to digest milk or milk products, is common in both Cambodians and Laotians.

TRADITIONAL HEALTH CARE BELIEFS AND PRACTICES

Self-medication and treatment may tend to be more common among Cambodians and Laotians than in many other Canadian residents. Few homes are without Tiger Balm, a mentholated ointment, which is used to treat a variety of conditions including colds, upset stomach, bruises, and insect bites. It is believed that some people may be allergic to the ointment. Medicines made from fresh herbs are used widely in home countries, but not in Canada, as the ingredients are not easily obtainable. The drinking of tonics, such as ginseng, and the avoidance of excess are common ways of maintaining health.

Many Cambodians and Laotians use a traditional practice known as coin rubbing in which an area of the body is rubbed with a metal object, usually a coin or spoon, until the skin becomes red. The area may be massaged first with a mentholated ointment, such as Vicks VapoRub or Tiger Balm, or with baby oil. This practice is commonly used to treat headaches, colds, fever, stomach-aches, dizziness, and fatigue. Different areas of the body are rubbed depending on the symptom or problem. For example, in the case of headache, the neck and forehead are usually rubbed. Coin rubbing is a common home remedy which continues to be used widely in Canada and is generally used when symptoms first appear and before a doctor is consulted. If the problem persists or is particularly troublesome, medical attention is usually sought. Another traditional treatment practised in Canada is the pinching of the skin between the eyebrows until it becomes red. This is used as a remedy for headaches and dizziness. Both coin rubbing and pinching cause bruising of the treated areas and when used on children can be mistaken for evidence of child abuse.

Most Cambodians from rural areas have consulted traditional healers or "loke kruu" in the past. These practitioners are greatly revered and trusted in rural society and are missed by many Cambodians living in Canada.

RELATIONSHIP BETWEEN PATIENT AND PROFESSIONAL

Typically, in Cambodian and Laotian cultures, the role of the health professional is authoritarian while that of the patient is passive and dependent. The professional is expected to ascertain quickly what is wrong, and the cure, or disappearance of symptoms, is expected to be fairly rapid. Doctors are highly respected and trusted members of society.

At a medical consultation a patient expects to receive some medication or treatment. For the doctor or health professional to suggest that there is nothing seriously wrong and that the condition will heal by itself is unacceptable. Most Cambodian and Laotian patients would be left feeling that the physician is uncaring and unhelpful. Similarly, being given tests before treatment is prescribed is meaningless to many people as it is not seen as part of the therapeutic process. Health professionals in Cambodia and Laos typically view the psychological support afforded to their patients as an important part of their healing role. The provision of some type of medication or treatment is regarded as integral to this support. "Placebos are widely used by practitioners in Southeast Asia in recognition of patients' expectation of receiving medicine and their usefulness in establishing rapport with a patient" (Muecke 1983:34).

Lack of fluency in English is a major problem for most Cambodians and Laotians in obtaining satisfactory care from health professionals in Canada. Unlike some other immigrant groups there are no professionals who speak their native languages in most areas of the country. It becomes necessary to rely on interpreters or on broken English, a less than satisfactory arrangement. Those fortunate people who can communicate in Vietnamese, Chinese, or French are sometimes able to consult practitioners who speak these languages.

Women prefer female physicians, especially for obstetrics and gynaecology. However, in Canada, most have male doctors and may thus be reluctant to discuss complaints and undergo regular check-ups. A Cambodian woman quoted her elderly mother as saying, "I'd rather die than be examined by a doctor who is a man."

Many Cambodians and Laotians in Canada only see a doctor when they feel seriously ill. This reluctance to seek early medical attention may stem from language difficulties and discomfort at the cultural differences that divide patient and professional.

MENTAL HEALTH

Mental illness is stigmatized by Cambodian and Laotian cultures; an individual who has mental health problems brings disgrace and shame to his or her family. As a consequence, mental illness tends to be feared and denied. Not infrequently people suffering from mental health problems are sheltered and hidden by family members until they can no longer cope. At that point they may seek professional help. Mental illness may be attributed to evil spirits by those with rural backgrounds or to karma by some Buddhists, that is, to the consequences of bad deeds committed in a previous life.

In Southeast Asian culture, where stoicism is a virtue and emotional weakness is unacceptable, "somatic complaints represent a cultural means of expressing psychological and emotional distress" (San Duy Nguyen 1984: 88). Cambodians and Laotians with mental health problems are likely to display a variety of physical symptoms, such as headaches, insomnia, aches and pains, fatigue, and dizziness. Because complaints are somatic, people tend to seek help from medical practitioners rather than mental health professionals, and they generally expect to receive medication.

Most mental health problems among Cambodians and Laotians in

Canada are linked to severe loss, the difficulty of cultural adjustment and uncertainty about the future. Refugees have typically gone through many traumatic experiences in rapid succession with little time to adjust. Often it is only after they have begun to settle into their new environment that the full impact of the losses and experiences is felt. Some may suffer "survivor guilt"; they may feel that they have no right to be alive or to live well when other family members and compatriots have died. Added to the stresses rooted in the past are those of the present: culture shock, language difficulties, social isolation, financial problems, and un- or underemployment. It is not surprising that depression is one of the most common mental health problems found in Southeast Asian refugees.

TREATMENT AND MEDICATION

It is commonly held among Cambodians and Laotians in Canada that North American medicine is too strong for them and that they are likely to suffer side-effects such as dizziness and even death. One Cambodian living in Canada reported, "Some people died in Cambodia after the Red Cross sent medicine from America." A contrary view held by others is that Western medicine is not strong enough. People of this persuasion have been known to increase the strength and frequency of the prescribed dosage. For example, a person who is told to take an antibiotic capsule four times a day might take two capsules each time, or take them five times a day.

There is a widely held belief in the effectiveness of injections over other forms of treatment. People who hold this view are likely to feel discouraged about the prospects for cure if only pills are prescribed.

Some fear blood tests, believing that the loss of blood causes dizziness and fatigue. Especially when in a weakened state, for example following surgery, people may feel that a blood test is actually life threatening and they may therefore need considerable reassurance before they consent. Cambodians and Laotians generally dislike and distrust invasive procedures such as surgery and post mortems and it is important that a need for these procedures be carefully and clearly explained.

Many people will often try traditional medicines and treatments at home before they seek help from a health professional. If symptoms do not improve medical attention is generally sought. Traditional treatments and medicines, such as herbal infusions, may be continued in conjunction with prescribed biomedical treatment without the physician being informed. A patient may appear to agree to a prescribed treatment and then not comply, or may behave

in a manner that effectively undermines it. Lack of compliance may
be due to disappearance of symptoms or to the influence of family or
friends. It is important to realize that in addition to the patient and
the immediate family, others may be involved in decisions about
treatment. "Extended family members, respected friends, and refugee leaders may all be participating by offering advice and caution-
ary guidance" (Pickwell 1983: 89).

HOSPITALIZATION

In Cambodia and Laos family involvement with a hospitalized
patient is extremely important. Generally speaking, the entire family is expected to visit daily. In Cambodia, a relative usually stays in
the same room with the patient and helps to care for him or her. In
both countries, visitors bring food and are encouraged to do so. In
many cases, meals are brought in as substitutes for hospital food.

In Cambodia, the physician usually visits a hospitalized patient
twice daily, and Cambodians in Canada may interpret the relative
infrequency of contact with their doctor as lack of concern.

Rural immigrants who have not had ready access to hospitals may
view them as places where one goes to die, since that is in fact what
often happens at home. For this reason, they are likely to fear and
avoid hospitalization in Canada.

Most Cambodians and Laotians are familiar with the idea of sign-
ing consent forms although many are likely to need an interpreter to
explain the details in each case.

Lack of fluent English is a major problem for the majority of Cambodians and Laotians hospitalized in Canada. The inability to communicate with hospital staff makes the experience frightening and
lonely. Many miss the traditional close support of family members.
Differences in food create a further difficulty; most Southeast Asians
eat rice three times daily and generally do not eat bread, potatoes,
cheese, butter, or milk.

FAMILY PLANNING

In rural areas of Cambodia and Laos families generally tend to be
large by Canadian standards with four to six children being the rule.
In these areas, birth control is usually not used, nor commonly
known. Among the urban population, the preferred methods of contraception are birth control pills and the IUD. In refugee camps,
women often had injections of Depo-Provera and may request it
here in Canada. Others who experienced side-effects with these

injections may refuse birth control pills. Many women have previously not taken continuous, on-going, daily responsibility for birth control. Some will choose tubal ligation once families are complete. In general, there is no special preference for the sex of offspring; both boys and girls are equally welcome.

In Canada, most Laotian and Cambodian couples prefer smaller families, with two or three children being the norm. There is a prevailing feeling that child-rearing is more expensive here and that a smaller family gives children a better chance of gaining a good education.

In the case of an unwanted pregnancy in Canada, a Laotian or Cambodian couple may decide on abortion.

PREGNANCY AND PRENATAL CARE

Cambodian and Laotian prenatal customs vary with ethnicity, region, rural and urban domicile, socio-economic background, and level of education. Some Cambodian women believe, for example, that hard physical work during pregnancy will result in easier delivery. Others hold that alcohol can be beneficial. For example, one notion is that beer consumption during pregnancy will lend the baby a beautiful, clear skin. Another is that an easy delivery will be assured if the mother imbibes a traditional white wine containing medicinal herbs when she is seven or eight months pregnant. There is a traditional Laotian belief that a pregnant woman should not attend a funeral nor visit anyone who has had a recent death in the family. Because practices vary, it is essential that health professionals find out from individual women what they believe to be important in their prenatal care.

In Cambodia and Laos when a woman becomes pregnant she first tells her husband and then her immediate family. It is happy news and pregnancy is considered a normal, healthy period in a woman's life. Only those living in urban areas receive regular medical attention. In Canada, some, but not all, Laotian and Cambodian women are interested in attending prenatal classes.

CHILDBIRTH

In Cambodian and Laotian cultures, the birth of a child is an occasion for celebration and ceremony. In rural areas, childbirth is generally at home. The mother and newborn are attended by a midwife who usually stays for three or four days following the birth. In urban centres, childbirth is generally in a hospital and a female member of a woman's family may stay with her during the period of hospitalization.

Traditionally the father does not participate in the birth, although in Canada some Cambodian and Laotian men may wish to support their wives by being present in the delivery room. Women who have already given birth in their home countries may feel uncomfortable delivering in a Canadian hospital because of the contrasts. In Laos, for example, as soon as a woman delivers, she must drink hot water; she should definitely not consume anything cold. There is a general fear of invasive procedures such as Caesarean section and episiotomy, and the need for such measures should be carefully explained. Circumcision is not typical. Young women who have not experienced childbirth may need some reassurance and explanation in order to understand the Canadian system but generally they do not have much difficulty.

POSTPARTUM PERIOD

According to both Cambodian and Laotian traditional beliefs, it is extremely important for women to keep warm after childbirth and many find Canadian hospitals too cold. After giving birth in rural areas of Cambodia, the woman rests on a special bamboo bed under which a charcoal fire is kept burning for up to a week. Windows may be closed and a woman usually covers her head. Cambodians also traditionally believe that women must not take showers or cut their hair for the first month postpartum; a woman washes in a mixture of warm water and a special wine which is believed to have medicinal properties. Laotian women traditionally take hot baths and drink warm fluids for twenty-one days to a month following birth. Many traditional beliefs and customs continue to be practised in Canada and need to be recognized and respected by health professionals. One woman told the story of a Cambodian woman who, after giving birth in a Canadian hospital, refused to take a shower. She finally gave in, however, at her husband's insistence and then fainted in the shower.

For the first month postpartum in Cambodia and Laos women are expected to stay at home and rest in bed while family members help with household tasks. Couples usually abstain from sexual relations for three months. Women generally breast-feed for up to a year and sometimes two years in rural areas. In Canada, some may choose to bottle-feed either because they have to return to work or because they feel it is more acceptable.

CHILDHOOD HEALTH AND ILLNESS

Common childhood diseases in Cambodia and Laos include dysentery and malaria. It is not uncommon for a six- or seven-year-old child to have an enlarged spleen as a result of periodic bouts of malaria. In refugee camps children were intensively immunized, but typically lack mumps and rubella vaccinations when they arrive in Canada. Parents may have been told that their children's immunizations were complete and may therefore need to be convinced of the need for more.

Children may suffer from anxiety and sleep disturbances caused by traumas experienced in their home countries and during escape, as well as by family separation and cultural adjustment.

In rural Cambodia and Laos children are usually treated for minor illnesses at home with traditional medicines and remedies, usually prescribed by grandparents. In Cambodia, TigerBalm or an equivalent ointment is routine treatment for infants and young children to prevent stomach-aches and relieve gas. This is rubbed on the child's stomach two to three times a day, especially after bathing and before bedtime. In Canada, because medical care is inexpensive and accessible, Cambodian and Laotian families are generally prompt in seeking medical attention for sick children.

FOOD AND NUTRITION

The traditional staple of the Laotian diet is a glutinous variety of rice which is steamed, while Cambodians eat standard rice. In addition fish, poultry, beef, pork, vegetables, and fruit are common items. Milk and milk products do not feature in the traditional diet and are generally disliked. In Canada, people prefer to retain traditional dietary habits and are able to find many of the necessary spices and ingredients in Chinese food stores. There may be an increased consumption of junk food, especially among children. Food is usually eaten with forks and spoons but sometimes with chopsticks.

Food preferences or taboos may be practised during periods of illness. Cambodians believe, for example, that stomach-ache sufferers should not eat fresh vegetables or oily food nor drink orange juice or anything acidic. Some Cambodians maintain that any type of skin disease or problem requires avoidance of beef, chicken, bamboo shoots, and eggplant. There may be people who prefer not to eat at all when they are sick.

Traditional food restrictions may also obtain during the perinatal period. A traditional Laotian belief, for example, requires that a new mother should avoid soup and spicy food and should eat only dry food. During the postpartum period, some Cambodian women may avoid beef, chicken, and raw vegetables. Because of the diversity of dietary beliefs and practices, it is necessary for the health professional to determine what the individual patient holds to be important in his or her health care.

ALCOHOL AND TOBACCO

In home countries, alcohol, most commonly traditional rice wine, is consumed by men. Use of alcohol by women, especially young unmarried women, is generally considered improper. Alcoholism is extremely rare. In Canada, Laotian and Cambodian men drink socially at parties or with visitors in the home; women, although consuming less than men, are more likely to accept alcohol here.

While many Cambodian and Laotian men smoke cigarettes, few women do so.

DENTAL PRACTICES

In Cambodia and Laos, dental care exists only in urban centres. Personal dental hygiene is generally good and teeth are cleaned daily. In rural areas, salt or lemon is frequently used in place of toothpaste. The poor nutrition experienced by many Cambodian and Laotian refugees as a result of shortages in their home countries and in the camps has contributed to gum and teeth problems.

CARE OF THE ELDERLY

In Cambodia and Laos, heart disease and cancer, including breast and uterine cancer, are less common among the aged than in Canada. There are no nursing homes or care facilities as families are expected to provide care for the elderly. In Canada these immigrants continue to honour their traditional responsibility. For example, a daughter would rather quit her job to care for an aged parent than allow him or her to be placed in a nursing home. To do otherwise would invite censure from the community.

DEATH AND DYING

For Cambodians and Laotians who are Theravada Buddhists, funeral is by cremation. Those who are ethnic Chinese bury their deceased, and those who are Christian converts arrange appropriate funeral services.

In Cambodia and Laos, according to the Theravada Buddhist belief, the deceased's body is washed and placed in a casket in the home. A wake is held for three days and nights during which family and friends visit, food and drink are provided, and the atmosphere is generally festive. On the third day, the body is taken to a temple where cremation takes place. On every anniversary of the death, family and friends participate in a memorial ceremony.

A person who knows that he or she is dying may request the family to gather so that last wishes may be expressed and belongings bequeathed to family members. Traditionally, Cambodians and Laotians prefer to die at home if at all possible. In home countries, a hospitalized patient who is terminally ill is often discharged so that he or she can return home to die.

ATTITUDE TOWARDS PUBLIC HEALTH AND SOCIAL SERVICES

Because there are no social services in Cambodia and Laos, immigrants to Canada from these countries may not understand their purpose, or know how to use them. Home visits by social workers may be accepted, but many people are unlikely to understand the relationship or know how to respond since involvement by strangers in personal matters is a foreign notion.

Young women are generally anxious to receive information and help from public health nurses about nutrition and infant care as many do not have older female family members in Canada to educate and assist them.

PROVIDING CULTURALLY SENSITIVE HEALTH CARE

In relating to immigrants from Cambodia and Laos formality and politeness are essential as they are a basic cultural expectation in clinical encounters. A slower pace and a quiet, unhurried manner are likely to reassure patients and will be more successful in establishing rapport and trust. Above all, it is necessary to recognize that Cambodians and Laotians are not a homogeneous group. Considerable diversity exists based on ethnicity, rural or urban background, level of education, and degree of exposure to Western health care. It is only through approaching patients as individuals that health care can be truly sensitive and appropriate to cultural and personal needs.

FURTHER READING

Asia Survey, Hong Kong, *Far Eastern Economic Review*, 1973–88

Background paper on the Laotian, Cambodian, and Hmong Refugees. City of Vancouver Task Force, Jan. 1980

Catanzaro, Antonio and Robert John Moser. "Health Status of Refugees from Vietnam, Laos, and Cambodia," *JAMA*, Vol. 247, No. 9 (5 Mar. 1982):1303–8

Chan, Kwok B. and Doreen Marie Indra, eds. *Uprooting, Loss, and Adaptation: The Resettlement of Indochinese Refugees in Canada*. Ottawa: Canadian Public Health Association 1987

Garry, Robert. "Cambodia," in Elliot Tepper, *Southeast Asian Exodus: From Tradition to Resettlement*. Ottawa: Canadian Asian Studies Association 1980

Indra, Doreen. "Khmer, Lao, Vietnamese, and Vietnamese-Chinese in Alberta," in *Peoples of Alberta: Portraits of Cultural Diversity*, ed. Howard and Tamara Palmer. Saskatoon: Western Producer Prairie Books 1985

Kiljunen, Kimmo. *Kampuchea: Decade of Genocide*. London: Zed Books 1984

Muecke, Marjorie A. "In Search of Healers: Southeast Asian Refugees in the American Health Care System," *Western Journal of Medicine*, 139 (Dec. 1983):835–40

Oberg, Charles N. and Amos Deinard. "Marasmus in a 17-Month-Old Laotian: Impact of Folk Beliefs on Health," *Pediatrics*, Vol. 73, No. 2 (Feb. 1984):254–7

Pickwell, Sheila M. "Nursing Experiences with Indochinese Refugee Families," *The Journal of School Health* (Feb. 1983):86–91

Royle, Peter. "Laos: The Prince and the Barb," in Elliot Tepper, *Southeast Asian Exodus: From Tradition to Resettlement*. Ottawa: Canadian Asian Studies Association 1980

San Duy Nguyen. "Mental Health Services for Refugees and Immigrants," *The Psychiatric Journal of the University of Ottawa*, Vol. 9, No. 2 (June 1984)

Tepper, Elliot L. *Southeast Asian Exodus: From Tradition to Resettlement*. Ottawa: Canadian Asian Studies Association 1980

Tung, Tran Minh. Indochinese Patients: Cultural Aspects of the Medical and Psychiatric Care of Indochinese Refugees. Washington, DC: Action for Southeast Asians, Inc. 1980

CONTRIBUTORS

Anhaouy Chansokhy (Immigrant Services Society, Vancouver)
Kate Frieson (Monash University, Melbourne, Australia)
Soma Ganesan (Vancouver General Hospital)
Nay Sim Ke (Vancouver)
Heng Khauv (Vancouver)
Madeline Lovell (UBC)
Lily Tham Phranchanah (Vancouver)
Banh T. Prom (Vancouver)
Sokhom Puth (Vancouver)
Donna Schareski (Vancouver Health Department, Burrard Unit)
T.K. Sihalathavong (Burnaby)
Duang Thavonesouk (Langley)
Khamvanh Xaygnachack (Langley)

CHAPTER THREE

The Central Americans

Danica Gleave and Arturo S. Manes

Forming a geographical arc between North and South America, Central America encompasses all the countries and cultures from southern Mexico to Panama. Since 1980, Canada has experienced a marked increase in the number of immigrants from this region, nearly all of whom have come as refugees. El Salvador, Guatemala, and Honduras are the most important countries of origin, with Nicaragua a distant fourth, although in many cases, people have come via Mexico or the United States. While the details of individual source countries are important in understanding why people have left for Canada, all the countries in the region, such as El Salvador, Guatemala, and others share a similar heritage and social conditions.

Spanish, English, French, and Dutch explorers began arriving some 400 years ago and made a lasting impact on the native population of the region. The sometimes violent introduction of Christianity, foreign languages such as Spanish, the contemporary Spanish semi-feudal landownership patterns as well as a host of other practical and intellectual devices from clothing to food caused major cultural shifts for the native people in the region. While many Indian communities succumbed to the new ways and disappeared, others were able to maintain their languages and customs, often incorporating European practices into their own cultures. The ancestors of Mayan people now living in rural Guatemala, for example, have combined a belief in Jesus Christ and other Christian figures with their traditional faith in the spirits of the natural world. Consequently, in Central America today one finds a wide spectrum of different cultures, from urban Westernized European descendants to rural landlords of mixed ancestry to Mayan-descended labourers who speak an Indian language and live in a traditional manner.

The implication for health professionals is that they must ask their Central American patients about their backgrounds. Since every individual has a unique history and story of migration, stereotyped images serve no useful purpose and can cause pain to everyone involved.

The experience of being a refugee is in itself uniformly gruelling, and to be further taxed by the misguided assumptions of professional helpers only adds to the individual's burden. Remembering this will be a giant step towards the delivery of compassionate and effective care.

SITUATION IN THE REGION

If one ignores political boundaries it is easy to envisage the backbone of mountains that swings southeast from Mexico to join the Andean range in South America. North of the mountains are various minor ridges and flat plains, many of which are covered in dense jungle. Lakes both large and small are found throughout the diverse countryside, a source of pleasure and beauty to both residents and visitors. The year-round tropical climate means that people coming to Canada will be unfamiliar with snowy winter conditions. The mountainous and tropical terrains combine to limit the available agricultural land, while political and economic interests ensure that this arable land is used overwhelmingly for cash crop production but worked by landless labourers.

These farms are often huge, owned by international corporations or wealthy families. This regional pattern of land ownership has helped to create a society with wide gulfs between the very wealthy and the poor. While professional classes exist, they are small and relatively powerless compared to the wealthy above them and are outnumbered heavily by blue collar workers, labourers, and un- or underemployed people beneath them. This imbalance in resource distribution has meant that by Canadian standards, roads and communications are inadequate, education and health facilities are poor, and so on. In El Salvador, for example, it is a legal requirement that every child between the age of seven and twelve attend school, but there are not nearly enough places to accommodate the nation's children. Dysfunctions such as these, accompanied as they are by an all-encompassing poverty, have been a primary source of the endemic political unrest and civil war in the region throughout this century. A second factor has been the tendency for nations in the area to be ruled by military dictators, most of whom have been liberal in their use of armed force to restrain public debate and civil uprising. Set within this historical context, the current turmoil in Guatemala, El Salvador, and Nicaragua begins to make more sense.

EL SALVADOR

El Salvador (whose name translates as "The Saviour") is both the smallest and most densely populated of the Central American countries, and is the source of most refugees coming to Canada from the region. Although more industrialized than its neighbours, El Salvador has unemployment ranging well above 50 per cent in rural areas. National statistics also reveal the disparity between rich and poor, as 0.5 per cent of the population control 50 per cent of the national income. Most people are of mixed Spanish and Indian descent, and Spanish is the national language. Approximately 40 per cent of the people are illiterate. Life expectancy is sixty-three years and there is a high birth rate—factors which result in a young population and heavy demand for jobs and arable farm land. The coffee crop has fueled the economy this century, although there are other export commodities, including cotton and sugar. Beans, corn, and rice are the dietary staples for most, and dairy products and meat are enjoyed when possible. Fresh vegetables and fruits are relatively abundant, especially in rural areas.

Politically, El Salvador has a history of military dictatorships, fraudulent elections (1972, 1976, and 1982), and state-sanctioned terror. Although the elections of 1982 were hailed by many in North America as the beginning of healthy democracy and the end of political violence, President Duarte and his government moved slowly to implement real change. Considering the traditional strength of the military and the deep fear of the United States about communist revolution in the region, as well as his own connections with the wealthy Salvadorean upper class, Duarte's lack of success was not surprising. Opposing the government is a rebel force, and clashes between the two, as well as "clean-up" campaigns and simple acts of terror by the army, have cost over 30,000 lives since 1979. At the same time, violence combined with crippling poverty has forced more than 300,000 refugees to flee El Salvador. Increasingly, these refugees and victims of murder, torture, and kidnap, are ordinary members of the population and not specific opponents of the government. Rural peasant communities are frequent targets of intimidatory military campaigns intended to deter them from assisting the guerrilla insurgents. Guerrillas can also use violence to force peasants to support them. Rural people therefore face an acute dilemma.

Health care, as with other social services, varies greatly between rich and poor, and between urban and rural areas. Doctors and hospitals are rare in the countryside, while overcrowded and poorly supplied public clinics and hospitals are standard for the urban working class. The wealthy can afford excellent care on par with any European or North American equivalent.

GUATEMALA

While the circumstances and details are different, the situation for Guatemalans is very similar to that of the Salvadoreans. Except for a ten-year democratic respite between 1944 and 1954, Guatemala has been ruled by a succession of military dictators since 1838. A handful of wealthy families controls most of the land and economic activities, leaving insufficient arable land to feed the rest of the population adequately. Consequently land reform is a key political issue. Coffee is by far the most important export crop, and coffee plantations are worked primarily by Mayan-descended people. Unlike other Central American countries, Guatemala has a large (53 per cent) population of native people, many of whom do not speak Spanish and remain virtually unassimilated into the urban culture. Over 50 per cent of the population is illiterate, life expectancy is fifty-seven years, and unemployment is chronic. As in El Salvador and other Third World countries, Guatemala has experienced major migrations from rural to urban areas as people come in search of jobs and services. Publicly funded hospitals, only available in the cities, are also overworked and understaffed.

As in El Salvador, state sponsored violence has been rampant. Since 1980, 50,000 people have been killed. Although a civilian president was elected in 1986, and political killings dropped briefly after the election, 1987 saw a renewal of these brutal tactics. The United States has invested heavily in Guatemala, and sends both economic and military aid. There are many restrictions on publishing, broadcasting, and group organization (Calvert 1985).

NICARAGUA

The current situation in Nicaragua is markedly different from Guatemala and El Salvador, although until recently their histories have shared elements in common. In 1979 the Sandinista National Liberation Front led and won a fight to topple Anastasio Somoza, whose family had held power since 1930. In taking Somoza property, the revolutionary government has brought 50 per cent of arable land

into public production. Despite an ongoing civil war, the legacy of a
$1.6 billion national debt, American import embargoes, and the
inherent traditional problems of high illiteracy and rural dispersion,
the Sandinistas have made substantial gains in implementing health
and education programs. The objective has been to bring health
professionals and facilities to the rural areas, and to integrate active
and interested locals into a preventive health care system.

More controversial has been the Nicaraguan government's
response to the Misquito Indians, resident in the northwest corner
of the country. Disappointed in their dealings with the Sandinistas,
and alarmed by government efforts to relocate them, many Misquito
have fled as refugees into neighbouring Honduras, where some have
joined the American-backed contra fighters.

Others who are non-native have left Nicaragua for North America
due to profound differences in political belief with the left-wing
government (and occasional bad treatment at the hands of the Sandinistas), or in fear of their lives because of the ongoing civil war.
Within the Central American communities in Canada, these ideological differences can sometimes create a gulf between Nicaraguans
and other refugees.

MIGRATION TO CANADA

Most immigrants from Central America have come as refugee claimants. A refugee is someone who is compelled to leave his or her home
for reasons of pressing personal safety and well-being. The person
concerned may have heard that he or she was on a new government
"hit list," may have witnessed the abduction or murder of friends
and family, or may have had their home and crops destroyed by the
military. They may also have experienced detention and torture.

There are three types of refugees. One group comprises politically
active opponents of the current regime who are forced into exile in
fear for their lives. Often middle-class professionals, these people
feel a strong bond with the home country and hope to return in the
future. A second group is the rural peasant population, whose
homes may be under general attack, and who flee to neighbouring
countries or regions for shelter. Often a whole village, consisting
primarily of women, children, and the elderly may move. These
people also hope to return home, and are often the beneficiaries of
international resettlement schemes to establish them as subsistence
agriculturalists in the host country.

Most refugees coming to Canada fall into the third group. These
are people who have not been active politically, although they may

have been members of a trade union or a similar organization. They are generally urban working class people or labourers who are able to gather the means to move northwards to the U.S. or Canada. These people, often single men, are nostalgic for the ways of home, but wish to settle and become established in Canada.

For many people the road to Canada is an indirect one, with lengthy stops in Mexico, Honduras, and, more commonly, the United States. Until February 1987 it was fairly easy for illegal residents in the U.S. to find jobs, and several people set up home and had children while there. For them, migration has meant not only leaving the original community in Central America, but also leaving the new home in the U.S. These people have the advantage of at least having more exposure to North American customs, food, expectations, and so on and, most importantly, have had the chance to learn some English.

The social, psychological, and economic implications of being a refugee affect every individual deeply and uniquely. As the later discussion of medical care for Central Americans will show, the immigration experience affects all aspects of a person's physical and mental health.

THE IMMIGRANTS

In the early 1980s when the first Central Americans began to come to Canada in any number, young working class men who were single or who had left their wives behind were the most common element. Recently there has been an increase in the number of families, most of which are fairly young. Elderly people are rare. The total Central American population in the Greater Vancouver region is estimated at between 4,000 and 5,000 and this number is growing. Both rural and urban people come, although the latter are the most common, and urban areas are more attractive as destinations in Canada. Many of these people have spent up to three or four years living and working in the U.S., gaining experience and skills that are valuable when seeking work here. A significant minority is illiterate in Spanish, which makes the task of learning written English very difficult.

The shock of being in Canada can last anywhere from one to three years, as people learn the language, have their immigration status finalized, establish a home in the new community, find jobs, and so on. When people apply for refugee status (which when successful results in landed immigrant status), they are screened for health problems, and if their initial application is not refused, are entitled to hardship assistance (a minimum amount of money for food and rent, e.g. in the summer of 1987 a young single man received $350 per month in Vancouver). After further processing, which usually takes a month or two, the claimant is allowed to make a statement under oath about the truth of his or her story. After this, the refugee is permitted to accept employment offers. Special papers are required for this, thereby lengthening the bureaucratic process.

While community and church groups, as well as concerned individuals, put tremendous amounts of time, energy, and money into sponsoring refugees or helping them to adjust to life in Canada, the bureaucratic immigration process leaves no refugee claimant unscarred. These immigrants, who worked hard at their jobs and were active in family and community life in Central America, are extremely unhappy about accepting charity and being seen as burdens to Canada. For example, although claimants recognize their legal entitlement to monetary support during the initial investigations, dealing with seemingly hostile and suspicious Department of Immigration and Employment clerks and queuing to collect cheques is frequently a humiliating process. For those refugees accepted while still outside the country, the federal government provides resettlement services such as furniture allowances. But this process involves obtaining a requisition from the Department of Immigration and Employment which entitles the holder to a selection of articles from the Army and Navy store. Someone at the store generally chooses the sofas, chairs, and so on which the refugee will receive. Although individual clerks both inside and outside the government have been caring and helpful, the system seems to discourage general compassion.

An assumption common to many Central American countries exacerbates this problem; namely, scepticism that fair and equal service can be expected from anonymous officials or professionals. In their communities of origin, these people usually did business and were served by extended, well-known groups, most of whose members were family. For example, unlike in Canada, an apartment or house would be found through social and family contacts. Or in a bank or other public office, one would only deal with staff known to the family. Experience has taught these people that services provided by persons unconnected with the family are worthless or even damaging. Initial guidance about Canadian procedures may help to alleviate misunderstanding.

Once a claimant can find and accept a job, many initial adjustment problems begin to be resolved. Although lack of English fluency often means that jobs are low-paying or menial, self-esteem improves, in that the person no longer feels like an object of charity. Both men and women look for work, and even though small children may prevent a mother from leaving the home, it is the women who are often more successful in finding initial employment. This can provoke extreme anxiety in husbands who are accustomed to being the family bread-winner. Typical jobs for both sexes include house-cleaning, dish-washing in restaurants, cutting and sewing in factories, cleaning windows, and so on. Some immigrants find that their initial digit "9" in their social insurance number deters potential employers and complicates the task of finding jobs.

While happy to work, middle-class professional refugees can become bitter about the marked decline in income and social status that is associated with the available jobs. Highly skilled, and often very experienced, these people are suddenly no longer valuable and esteemed. For many there is little hope of resuming their careers in Canada. For example, immigrant physicians will not receive the necessary residency training in hospitals even if they pass the qualifying exams. This is particularly frustrating, given the media reports about the lack of medical services in northern and rural Canada. They have the skills and the willingness to go to these areas but are prevented from doing so.

LANGUAGE

For nearly all Central American immigrants the primary obstacle to getting settled, finding jobs, and obtaining satisfactory medical care is the lack of ability in English. Those accepted outside the country as bona fide refugees under the federal assistance program, are entitled to five months of free English classes. But others (the great majority) who come independently to the border to seek refugee status are only provided with funding for food and shelter. Church groups, school boards, concerned volunteers, and some public libraries offer free or very inexpensive classes. However, even after six months or so of instruction, many people still lack the confidence to accept jobs requiring English proficiency, or even to participate fully in the life of the larger Anglo-Canadian community. As one woman observed, "Language is the biggest thing. People think they're never going to learn English, it's so hard."

For women with children, the pressures of having to go to classes and finding child care on a very limited budget can lead to depression.

EXPERIENCE WITH CANADIANS

Central American refugees overall are deeply grateful to Canada for the aid and shelter provided, but language difficulties as well as financial restrictions are the main obstacles to developing friendships with many Canadians. In Vancouver and other large urban centres there is a large enough community of fellow Spanish-speaking immigrants to provide companionship and help. The overwhelming support given by the community to needy members speaks volumes for the group's generosity and compassion. However, in terms of social life, the predominantly working class Central Americans do not associate with the professionals who came as political refugees from Chile and Argentina in the 1970s, despite their common language.

SPECIAL PROBLEMS IN CANADA

While Central Americans do not share the problems of traditional dress or physical features experienced by some other immigrant groups, racism is at times a considerable problem. Lack of English, darker skin tones, and poverty can give rise to bigoted accusations of stupidity, laziness, and so on.

A domestic problem for many people is the role change between husband and wife after they come to Canada. In Central America the man traditionally has the responsibility of providing for the family's material needs. He also has a widely accepted privilege of establishing long-term mistresses and second families. Wives have not welcomed these arrangements, but they are accepted as the status quo because limited employment opportunities for women make a man's financial contributions essential. Wives have the traditional responsibilities of the home, bearing and raising children, cooking, cleaning, maintaining health care, and so on. Once in Canada, it is soon recognized that opportunities exist for women to raise their status, and so threaten the man's position. When wives are the first to find work, husbands may experience depression. Sometimes men may even discourage their wives from learning English or, in severe cases, may resort to violence. In the latter instance, the woman's entitlement to police protection and legal redress here may shock the husband even further and be seen as a direct challenge to his marital rights. Support, counselling, and an explanation of the Canadian notions of basic human rights, can help to resolve these difficulties.

Problems can also arise between generations. Some of the few elderly people who have come to Canada, feel that they are no longer seen as sources of family knowledge and have consequently lost the deep respect that they enjoyed in Central America. Instead they feel ill used, and have become mere live-in baby-sitters and house cleaners.

Raising teenagers in Canada presents a host of difficulties in addition to the normal stresses of adolescence. While boys in Central America are allowed considerable freedom and have few domestic responsibilities, girls are not permitted to stay out late, to date and associate with whom they please, and so on. They also cook, clean, and care for younger siblings. To Central American parents the life of the urban Canadian teenager appears to be filled with reckless abandon. Working out some kind of satisfactory compromise within the family therefore becomes difficult. In extreme cases parents can feel betrayed by the government when social services provide their children who have moved away from home with welfare money for rent and food. They believe strongly that they know what is best for their children.

During the early years of life in Canada, children are also often the first to learn English, an ability they have been known to use as a source of power over their parents. Some parents are shocked by the behaviour and values of Canadian teenagers, and think these to be a bad influence on their own children, especially the girls.

RELIGION

While the statistics for Central America indicate that nearly everyone is Roman Catholic, there is considerable diversity among the immigrants reaching Canada. Many are active Catholics, who accept the church both as provider of social support and as a major participant in community life. In Central America, religious festivals mark the calendar much more strongly than in Canada, with such events as Carnival being celebrated as festive holidays.

Others are non-practising members of the church, with varying degrees of commitment to Catholic belief and ritual. Many are Protestants, either by birth or conversion. The aid given by particular church groups to refugees has resulted in some immigrants joining that church. Evangelization is also taking place with some success in Central America itself. The Mennonites, Jehovah's Witnesses, Mormons, and Baha'i are among those denominations which have Central American followers.

Although there are few Mayan-descended Guatemalan refugees in Canada, their religious beliefs probably combine traditional spiritual concepts with Christian ideas.

FAMILY STRUCTURE

When a couple marries, they are expected to set up an independent household which is intimately, though not physically, tied to the extended families on both sides. The husband is head of the family, but important decisions, including those concerning health care, will generally be made in consultation with the wider family. The number of children in a family may range from four to six, but the example of the smaller Canadian families around them causes these immigrants to restrict the size of their families.

In their home countries people from urban areas may be accustomed to having a maid to help with household chores.

The extended family is made up of both blood relatives and so-called fictive kin, such as godparents, creating a widespread net of social, business, professional, and bureaucratic connections. While godparents are essentially a Christian tradition, their role is important and serious in nearly all social aspects of a child's life. They have the right to offer advice to parents and are expected to care for the child in the event of the parents' death. Extra sets of godparents are added at communion and marriage, and will provide food and money for the celebrations. In El Salvador, for example, the bridal couple's godmother brings an elaborate, delicious cake, while the godfather gives the groom a pouch of silver coins with which to "buy" his bride. More importantly, godparents enlarge the communal links of trust and security for the couple and their children.

MARRIAGE AND DIVORCE

The pattern in Central America is for people to marry young compared to Canada. Women will be between sixteen and nineteen years of age, while men are in their early twenties. Virginity is considered important for women though not for men. Common law unions are rare and frowned upon as marriage is seen to provide legal security for the wife and children.

The frequency of divorce varies greatly between classes and religious groups. Affluent urban residents are believed to have more divorces than others. Practising Catholics, especially those living in rural areas, are far less likely to divorce, even in extreme situations. For women, the stigma of divorce can be a heavy burden, but some are willing to risk this rather than live with a man who is abusive or keeps a mistress. After divorce, the most common method of obtaining support is for the woman and her children to return to her family's home. The husband's family may also take responsibility for raising a child, especially a son.

WOMEN

When a baby is expected, the parents keenly anticipate either a boy or a girl, although their expectations for a child of either sex are not necessarily the same. As in other areas of the world, a girl will grow up with the paramount objective of becoming wife, mother, and home-maker. Naturally, every individual interprets these ideas differently, and a small but active feminist community in Central America is beginning to voice its opposition to the traditional roles and inequalities.

Customarily and ideally the woman's territory is the home, while men are responsible for activities away from the domestic sphere. For this work, women are theoretically esteemed and respected, but this can often lead to a false evaluation of status. While domestic labour undeniably involves hard physical work, long hours, and few monetary rewards, it is not esteemed as highly by either men or women as male wage labour. When people come to Canada it is regarded as demeaning as well as burdensome for a husband to take over child care duties if his wife is the first to find a paying job. Some women will even refrain from seeking outside work until their husbands are employed.

In the Central American countries of origin, general unemployment is very high, so that jobs for women are scarce, particularly well paid and respected jobs. Even if the financial resources are available they seldom pursue high school, technical, or university education, which limits their employment prospects even more. Instead financial security is sought in marriage, which is seen to hold the promise of support by the husband for his wife and children. This valuation is so strong that wives will tolerate their husband's mistresses, albeit uneasily. It also reinforces the husband's right to use physical force in arguments with his wife. Mistresses are also seeking economic support and by bearing a child with the man's name a financial claim is made on him. Situations have arisen in Canada where women in this position have wanted to give the baby its biological father's name. Careful explanation of Canadian law and customs is therefore called for.

The women's role in the home and community is a strengthening and enriching one, and it is often the women who hold the family together during the stresses of flight and relocation. Nonetheless, most women coming to North America enjoy a marked improvement in legal rights and social or work opportunities. This is certainly so for their daughters. As mentioned before, this change in status can exacerbate marital tensions.

For many women, the biggest problem faced in Canada, aside from financial and immigration worries, is isolation. Language barriers, physical distance, reserved Canadian neighbours, and busy North American schedules put limits on Central American-style casual hospitality. These women are used to tolerating a great deal of concern and anxiety, which they would not unburden on their mothers even at home. Isolation can come in many forms. One typical sorrow confronting women here is the knowledge that one or more children have been left behind in Central America. When parents leave their home countries, they do not always have sufficient resources to bring every child, either by way of money or the physical carrying power to walk to Mexico and swim the Rio Grande. They usually hope that money will be found quickly to bring the child north.

TABOO TOPICS

Sexuality is not generally or openly discussed, especially between members of the opposite sex, including a male physician alone with a female patient. Homosexuality in particular is taboo, although many Central Americans regard physical warmth between men as acceptable and desirable. Many people may be aware of the existence of homosexual men "in the city" but lesbianism is very much closeted.

CHILDREN

Children are universally welcomed and a large family is often a measure of status, especially in rural areas. While the parents, especially the mother, are the primary sources of care, the extended family shares in these responsibilities. Young children often spend their playtime roaming the streets in groups, visiting neighbours, and playing games. Bottle-feeding and disposable diapers will be used for infants whenever possible by immigrants from urban areas, as these are a sign of technological progress and financial status. Many women find the Canadian emphasis on breast-feeding confusing and unsettling, as the infant formula advertisements at home have emphasized the superior growth of bottle-fed babies. Child discipline is variable and there may be more physical aggression amongst the urban middle and upper classes than among rural families.

THE ELDERLY

At present there are very few elderly Central Americans in Canada, although as younger immigrants gain citizenship and begin to sponsor family members, this situation will change. Central America's life expectancies are low by Canadian standards, ranging from fifty-seven years in Guatemala to sixty-three years in El Salvador, and as in other parts of the world women outlive men.

There are no old people's homes in Central America. Rather, older members expect to live with or be cared for by younger generations in the family. Failure to provide care or shelter is a source of shame for the family. An older mother-in-law can be the focal point of a family, respected for the knowledge that a long life has given her. This situation, when transported to Canada has led to deep tensions, as the older woman's wisdom is no longer valued and she becomes a simple baby-sitter while her children go out to work. Learning English is particularly burdensome for these older people and they often see no point in making the effort. This in turn can exacerbate their social isolation.

NAMES

The customary naming system in Central America differs significantly from North America in that when a woman marries she both retains her father's name and takes her husband's. For example, if Maria Sanchez marries Juan Lopez, she becomes Maria Sanchez de Lopez. Her husband's name does not change. Their children will be, for example, Pedro Lopez Sanchez. Because the connecting "de" in a married woman's name means "belonging to" there are pockets of feminist resistance to its use.

Thus all elements in an immigrant family will have different last names, which can create bureaucratic confusion in Canada as well as hot tempers if questions are raised about the legitimacy of a marriage or child. Although some feel that the solution is for the family to take only the father's name, this can create problems for people returning to Central America since legal documents will not then be in acceptable order.

For a professional to call someone by his or her first name is seen as negative, and patronizing. This is because historically, landowners and other wealthy people have addressed their workers by using first names in the diminutive Spanish "tu" form, which is usually reserved for children and pets.

PATTERNS OF COMMUNICATION

Compared to Canadians, Central American people relish physical warmth and closeness. This is as true of members of the same sex as of mixed couples.

People generally show tremendous deference and respect to those in positions of authority such as physicians. At the same time, they feel uncomfortable about making immediate eye contact with strangers. Their lowered eyes should not be interpreted as lack of interest or docility, but rather as simple good manners.

Problems and sorrows often give rise to an apparent sense of fatalism. Misfortune is simply God's will and must be dealt with accordingly. In rare cases, this may for example prompt resistance to preventative health measures such as vaccination or diet changes. The assumption is that if the victim was meant to get diptheria or have a heart attack, then so be it.

SHOPPING

Women are responsible for shopping for the daily needs of the household. For them, the differences between the lively Central American markets and the anonymous supermarkets of North America can be enormous. Initially, women many need guidance on comparison shopping, reading labels, bargains, and so on. The immigrant Central American community will often rally to a woman's aid and help her find her way in the system. Husbands will be responsible for decisions on major purchases, although a wife will participate in the final choice of individual product.

TIME

The subject of many jokes, the Latin American sense of time is renowned for its flexibility. In practice in Canada, Central American respect for appointment times and deadlines varies among individuals. Many are very punctual, others less so. Explaining the importance of a health professional's timetable, and giving the assurance that the health professional will be on time, can help. It can also be useful to emphasize that the custom in Canada is to be punctual for appointments.

SLEEPING PRACTICES

Depending on the social stratum of the family, they may have slept in a single room or had separate bedrooms. In either case, once in Canada families quickly adjust to the idea that children sleep separately from their parents, although a baby is likely to share its parents' room.

RECREATION AND LEISURE

A significant difference in social life between Canada and Central America is the informal quality of visits and gatherings in El Salvador, Guatemala, and Nicaragua. While neighbours respect each other's privacy, doors are always open to the casual visitor who has time to spend chatting or sharing in a household task. A community will often have a few established meeting spots such as a park or bar where friends can be found during weekend afternoons or evenings. The custom of carefully arranging visits by phone ahead of time seems cool and stilted to many Central Americans.

Recreational activities depend largely on income levels, gender, and age, but group events are more likely to occur away from home. An extended family group may go to a restaurant, or young people may go to a disco, and so on. Men particularly enjoy watching and playing soccer, to the extent that in Vancouver the community has established nearly twenty teams. They may share a drink after a game, but otherwise alcohol has no particular social importance. Women may come together and cook their favourite dishes when preparing for a family feast. Trips to a lake or the ocean are real treats, and hiking excursions into the mountains are holiday specialities.

Differences in language and custom represent barriers between English-speaking Canadians and Central American immigrants, but when they do meet the experience is generally positive for both sides.

FESTIVALS AND HOLIDAYS

Roman Catholic celebrations throughout the year are the biggest and most popular holidays. These include familiar events such as Christmas, but others, such as Lent, have much greater significance for Central Americans. During Lent weekends carnivals, complete with games and cotton candy, are organized in church squares. Great efforts are made by congregations to enliven the churches with thousands of flowers, bountiful produce, music, and so on. Another important festival unusual in Canada occurs on November 2. This is a more sombre occasion, in which dead family ancestors are honoured. People speak warmly of these different festivals and miss them as part of the familiar community life that they enjoyed in Central America.

HEALTH CARE SYSTEMS IN CENTRAL AMERICA

The type and quality of care available in the region varies greatly with location and family income. Rural peasants and labourers have access to few Western-style medical personnel and facilities. For them, the traditional views of health and illness are much more valid than for their urban counterparts. However, they are receptive to the spread of scientific medical practices which they see as a sign of progress. The traditional approach is largely based on a classification of hot and cold qualities. Certain sicknesses and conditions are considered hot, others cold. Food and medicines also fall into these categories. To maintain good health, the object is to establish temperature equilibrium. Using this logic the treatment of a hot condition (i.e., fever) with a "hot" medicine (some antibiotics) will be seen as counterproductive. Generally, those people coming to Canada will have left most such ideas behind, but because they are basic health care principles and have been ingrained in every child, they are still occasionally apparent. Childbirth and the postpartum period are seen as very cold times, and sometimes new mothers in Canadian hospitals will be shocked to be served ham, a notoriously cold food.

In urban areas, money is the biggest deciding factor in the type of health care available. For the wealthy, there are private physicians and hospitals which provide care on par with international standards. For the majority, however, local lay specialists and underfunded, overcrowded public hospitals provide the bulk of the medical care. Although hospital conditions are generally poor, and stories abound of emergency patients having to make do with shots of valium and of wounds being sewn up with a dressmaker's needle and thread, people still go to the hospitals for help. It is considered much better to have a baby in hospital, for example, than at home with a midwife even though the hospital may be so crowded that women deliver standing up and there are no available recovery beds.

Regardless of education level or place of residence, Central Americans have an overwhelming knowledge of prescription drugs and the conditions for which they are appropriate. They will very often request a physician directly for a specific drug that they know to have been helpful in the past. Prescribing medication is an indication to the patient that he or she is being taken seriously and treated well.

On the other hand, there are considerable gaps in people's knowledge, especially among the poor and uneducated. For example, a concept as fundamental to Western medicine as germ theory is either unknown or dismissed by segments of the population. The argument is the familiar one—if you cannot see it, it does not exist.

Common home remedies that people bring to Canada include herbal teas and the use of Vicks VapoRub for headaches, feverish babies, and a multitude of other discomforts. People from rural areas often use herbal packs for ailments such as fever, but many of the plants they need are not available in Canada. Eucalyptus is widely and variously used. Coins may be placed on a newborn's umbilical cord to prevent hernias and the soles of a child's feet may be painted with a red mixture as a cure for infection.

PREVALENCE OF DISEASE

Since the immigration process weeds out people in poor general health, serious diseases are not common among Central Americans resident in Western Canada. There is often radiological evidence of inactive cases of tuberculosis. An occasional case of syphilis is found, but the incidence of other sexually transmitted diseases is about the same as for the general Canadian population, and may be lower for women.

Parasitic infections are widespread, if not universal, in this population and need attention. Evidence of torture, from broken legs to cigarette burns, is also not uncommon among Central Americans. Professionals specializing in rehabilitating torture survivors emphasize that the emotional damage is far greater than the physical injury. While physical wounds may heal the related psychological trauma may be so deep as to rule out the physician's raising the subject before the patient has broached it. Once a relationship of trust has been established, and this can take years, the patient may reveal his or her story. Until then it may be best to leave the subject untouched.

MENTAL HEALTH

Pregnancy and childbirth aside, mental health disorders and related physical problems are the most frequent cause of Central American contact with the Canadian health system. The experience of being a refugee, from initial persecution to flight away from family and friends to the host country, is gruelling and draining. People have great hopes that when they reach Canada, the problems such as poverty, malnutrition, and persecution will disappear. Instead they are faced with the tremendously stressful immigration process and lengthy waits for landed immigrant status, work permits, jobs, housing, and so on. Learning English is another major anxiety, especially for refugee claimants ineligible for sponsored language classes. These worries can lead to bitterness and anger, to the extent that some people declare they should have stayed at home and died fighting rather than be subjected to Canadian immigration procedures.

As time passes, the roles of husband and wife, parent and child begin to diverge from the models familiar in Central America. Many husbands are depressed in the early years in Canada as they see their traditional family position eroding.

For serious mental illness in Central America, people are institutionalized with the expectation that they will never recover or be discharged. The belief in the helpfulness of talking about problems with close family or friends is less clearly recognized by Central Americans. Spouses do not habitually discuss intimate topics with each other, but may respond well when the suggestion is made to them. Encouraging people to socialize and discuss their worries with friends can also be a help. Here, as in Central America, drugs are readily prescribed to treat depression and anxiety. Counselling in Canada can be difficult because of the language barrier and the lack of Spanish-speaking practitioners. The extent of the depression and its pervasive links with living conditions and life stresses also militate against effective counselling. As one woman noted: "It's difficult to counsel someone when everything can be a problem, even figuring out how to catch a bus to the Food Bank."

As people become settled, have their immigration status confirmed, and establish homes, jobs, and a place in the community, anxiety and depression fall away, as do the associated aches and pains.

RELATIONSHIP BETWEEN PATIENT AND PROFESSIONAL

Canada's medical system is so different from that in Central America that an important part of a health professional's initial role is to advise patients on the resources available and the functioning of the system. People come expecting that health care here will be better, more technologically advanced and, through health insurance, more accessible. However, the practicalities of the system are often unfamiliar and need explanation: things such as having a physician on call and a regular family doctor, well baby clinics, optometrists but not dentists, being covered by medical insurance coverage, and so on. Clearly encouraging patients to ask questions and request help as a right is also important. Some physicians have found that only 10 per cent of their time with a patient is used on diagnosis, the remainder being used for preventative education and information on the health care system.

The ideal model of interaction between physician and patient in Central America is as follows. The patient calls to see the doctor, who is either known or directly related to the patient's family. The physician takes a few minutes to discuss general unrelated topics, may walk around the room, guide the patient to a chair with a gentle arm around the shoulders, and so on. After the patient has been put at ease in this manner, the doctor takes a seat and listens very carefully to the patient's story. The physician is expected to take his client's concern seriously, to label the problem for the patient, and to prescribe suitable medication. (The patient in fact may already have a drug in mind.) Treatment of some kind—be it shots, tablets, or creams—is the patient's criterion for success. Doctors who do not prescribe drugs are considered very poor. It is also customary in some areas for a female relative to accompany a woman when she sees her male doctor. This is dictated by modesty and by the need to allay the husband's jealousy.

These expectations have several implications for Latin immigrants and their doctors. The idea that good care can be received from an anonymous doctor is initially foreign, and North American directness in medical interviews can aggravate the patient's uneasiness. The Canadian goals of limiting medication and performing comprehensive tests prior to treatment are welcomed by the general Canadian population, but have the opposite effect on Central Americans. Some new immigrants, treated in this manner and unable to communicate effectively with their doctor, have sworn that North American doctors "don't care" and "don't know their subject well enough to provide good treatment."

The idea that relaxation or exercise can help a problem can also be poorly received, as is revealed by the story of the woman who had a terrible headache. She went to Emergency for help, where she was examined and told that nothing was physically wrong and that she should simply go home to rest until the headache passed. Feeling misunderstood and poorly treated, she went away resentful and in pain. Careful explanation, and the assurance that the patient is being taken seriously, can help to alleviate these tensions.

Practical details needing clear discussion are the regular use of a general practitioner to attend to a family's health needs over a period of years. For those Central Americans who received all their care from clinics, a long-term relationship with one doctor is novel. The purpose of regular check-ups and test procedures such as pap smears, breast self-examinations, and prostate checks are generally unfamiliar, as is the theory of preventative medicine. People are interested and concerned about their health, so that taking the time to explain things clearly will be highly beneficial.

Some women patients may feel much more comfortable with a female physician. When this is not possible, the presence of a nurse or other woman in the room during an internal examination can be a great help. This should not be automatically presumed, however; one Vancouver doctor discovered that his female patients grew perplexed when he asked his nurse to come in. The patients felt their private business was becoming too public.

Central Americans will want to see a doctor when they have a concern, even though many of the problems appear minor to Canadian health professionals. A new mother may want to take her baby to the doctor whenever it gets a pimple, for example; or a slight rise in a child's fever at night can send parents quickly scurrying for help. The challenge for the physician is to avoid over-prescribing while still giving reassurance. Some physicians have found that as families adjust to life in Canada, the frequency of visits diminishes. The feeling is that people use physicians to confirm their well-being as much as to treat medical problems. As times passes the former need diminishes.

While doctors hold a similar place in terms of training and prestige in both Canada and Central America, nurses do not. There are very few professional schools for nurses in the region and most women receive their training on-the-job by working closely with a physician. While they are able to do more of the mundane work usually performed by physicians here, such as sewing wounds and so on, they are not respected as are Canadian nurses, but rather are seen as menial hospital workers. In places, notably Nicaragua, recent campaigns are aimed at boosting the status of nurses as health professionals and at enhancing their training to include community health work. However, nurses in Canada should be clearly introduced as professionals to new immigrants. The abilities of nurses and the services they provide, once demonstrated to newcomers, will confirm this status. Central Americans who have spent time in Canadian hospitals have generally been delighted with the skill and solicitude of nurses. As one woman noted, "The idea of being asked if I needed anything! This never happened to me at home in Guatemala." Public health nurses can be particularly helpful to immigrants in guiding them through the medical system and integrating them into the new community.

HOSPITALIZATION

Depending on a person's background, hospitalization in Central America can be associated with death rather than recovery. While these fears may linger on in some immigrants, most trust the capabilities, high standards, and objectives of hospitals here, and are, in one doctor's opinion, model hospital patients. Privacy, clothing, and food present no problems, apart from the postpartum food taboos concerning pork and other "cold" foods. Patients with fever may also resist bathing. Central American families tend to visit convalescing relatives more frequently and in larger groups than Anglo-Saxons, but not to a disruptive degree. Consent forms are a novelty and need translation as well as explanation. As in other aspects of health care, language barriers present the biggest problem. Although it is often difficult for people to be lucid, racism has also occasionally been felt. One example was a woman present in hospital for a prenatal examination. Despite her protests, she was subjected to a series of internal examinations by a group of medical students. This type of problem is not, of course, limited to Central Americans.

Post mortems are uniformly disliked unless absolutely necessary, the feeling being that the family member is already dead and should not be subjected to further trauma. Physicians will need exceptionally good arguments to overcome this sentiment.

MEDICATIONS AND TREATMENTS

Although the technology and the theory behind much North American medical treatment will be new to Central Americans, they generally perceive it as advanced and are willing to comply. Points of contention arise when doctors do not prescribe medication for a patient as this signifies that the physician is not taking the condition seriously. Some physicians work around this by giving simple vitamins or non-prescription drugs for symptomatic relief.

Testing before treatment is also unfamiliar and may be interpreted as lack of concern. For example, a family grew angry with the attending physician when their son was hospitalized for severe pains in his legs. The extensive tests were seen as experimental procedures on a human guinea pig, while nothing appeared to be done to alleviate the pain. Language problems exacerbated the problem, but the story illustrates a common Central American fear. Considering that drug companies have been known to undertake unethical testing of new products in the Third World, Central Americans have some historical grounds for their concerns about experimentation.

Central Americans will be as compliant as other groups about following a treatment schedule. As with others, there is a tendency to stop taking medication when symptoms disappear, thus necessitating clear prior instructions and explanations. Lack of money can prevent people from having a prescription filled. The complicated procedure laid down by the Department of Immigration and Employment to pay medical costs can be enough to prevent sick people from getting medication. There are Jehovah's Witnesses in the Central American group, and these people will refuse blood transfusions.

Common Canadian ideas about rehabilitation exercise will be unfamiliar to many Central Americans. They expect to spend the time in hospital inactively, convalescing. The encouragement of health professionals to get out of bed and exercise as soon as possible after surgery can be confusing and threatening. A Central American man who had hand surgery to correct a long-term, slightly crippling condition, could not believe the doctor who told him to start exercising and using the hand normally as soon as possible. When he disregarded suggestions, his hand became stiff and painful thereby reinforcing the patient's initial lack of faith in the surgeon. As a rule, however, people expect to recover fully and resume normal activities. When rehabilitation practices are explained as being a part of the process people have generally been very responsive.

THE DISABLED

Life for a person in Central America with either mental or physical disabilities depends greatly on the financial resources and social position of the family. In all cases, with the recent exception of Nicaragua, there are no public social services for the disabled, and their care is the responsibility of the family, although the patient will be loved and protected. Disabled people will not often appear in public, partly for fear of ridicule and insult and partly because there are no facilities or jobs for them. The exception to this for some poor families is that a disabled person may be sent out to beg, which may make all the difference to the family's financial survival.

Shortly before one family left Nicaragua a program was initiated for people in wheelchairs to play basketball. The family members recall their initial incredulity, and the delighted surprise which followed when the project turned out to be fun, exciting and popular. In short, like other people in Canada, Central Americans may initially doubt the abilities of disabled people.

FAMILY PLANNING AND SEXUALITY

For Central Americans, talking about sexuality and related subjects does not come as easily as for most Anglo-Canadians, although women are concerned enough about contraception to initiate the occasional discussion with their physicians. For problems of sexual dysfunction, such as premature ejaculation, men are much more likely than women to approach a doctor, although even here numbers are very small.

Knowledge about fertility can vary greatly along class, age, and gender lines, with large segments of the population being very ignorant of the biology of reproduction. For example, since virginity is an important ideal for unmarried women, some girls believe literally that pregnancy cannot occur before marriage, a mistake which can lead to many accidents. Education is clearly the solution.

Although Central American families tend to be larger than their average Canadian counterparts, wives are very interested in controlling their fertility. Birth control is seen as a "woman's problem" and methods which require male participation, such as condoms, are unlikely to be well received. Once again, differences exist, as one physician has Mayan patients who happily use both condoms and the Billings (rhythm) method! The pill is widely accepted, the IUD is tolerated but diaphragms are unpopular. Withdrawal is probably the most commonly used practical method.

In the event of unwanted pregnancy, about 50 per cent of women favour abortion, once they know it is legal procedure in Canada, and despite their strongly Roman Catholic backgrounds. Abortion is illegal throughout Central America, although many unlawful abortions are performed under often terrible circumstances. Frequently these illegal terminations result in sepsis, infertility, and even death. It is not unusual to find women who have undergone illegal abortions among the immigrants to Canada. However, it is important to note that the Spanish word for miscarriage and abortion is the same.

Although sexually transmitted diseases (STDs) are rare in refugees entering Canada, there are occasional cases of syphilis. In Central America itself, the rate of STDs may be very high relative to Canadian levels.

PREGNANCY

Class and geography determine the kind of prenatal care a woman experiences in Central America. For rural women, pregnancy and childbirth will be overseen by a local midwife, and mothers and other older women in the community will provide the necessary support, knowledge, and household help. For working class and poor urban women, the situation is similar except that they usually deliver in a hospital or polyclinic, even though they may have had no formal prenatal medical care. Rich urban women will use the best physician and hospital services available.

Prenatal classes are unheard of in Central America, although those classes offered in Spanish in Vancouver are well attended. Husbands need firm encouragement to go, but once they see the other male participants they make good-spirited efforts to take part. Since birth procedures in Canada are so unfamiliar, clear information on the working of the system as well as tours around the hospital are invaluable. For example, it can be helpful to mention to new immigrant women that it is not necessary to bring their own sheets with them to hospital.

Pregnancy is generally considered a healthy and happy time, but women are encouraged to take precautions against damaging the foetus. For example, the food cravings of an expectant mother must be satisfied to guard against birth defects.

CHILDBIRTH

Central American immigrant women's experience of childbirth in Canada has been very positive, despite the unfamiliarity of customs. Language presents the greatest problem, and often husbands have to translate. Fathers are not normally permitted into hospital delivery rooms in Central America, but with appropriate encouragement, many attend here. However, some women feel uncomfortable at the prospect and prefer to bring a female friend or relative. Health care workers should respect this choice.

New-born babies often have their waists tied with a belly band, or they have a coin placed on the umbilicus to prevent a hernia. While these practices may seem unnecessary to Western doctors or nurses, they bring peace of mind to the new parents. Infant sons will not be circumcised. Baby girls often have their ears pierced after two or three months, and if doctors refuse to do the piercing, parents will do it themselves or find someone else.

Women are familiar with Caesarean sections and generally accept whatever procedures the physician deems necessary to deliver a healthy baby. At the same time, they will tolerate considerable pain before asking for an anaesthetic.

POSTPARTUM PERIOD

The degree to which women follow traditional practices will dictate how much the postpartum period diverges from mainstream Canadian customs. Rural women new to North America are the most likely to observe the traditional forty-day postpartum period during which they ideally remain indoors, away from drafts, and with their head, ears, and feet covered. They are expected not to watch television or listen to the radio, to eat proper warming foods such as tortillas, and to avoid cold ones such as pork. Bathing is considered risky because of its potential for chilling the new mother. She will also wear a special girdle to prevent the uterus from becoming dislocated or, in more recent times, to aid its return to its original size. It must be remembered that these practices represent one end of the spectrum. Most women will retain what they consider to be the valuable parts of the tradition, while others dispense with custom altogether.

A major issue facing new mothers in Canada is the strong pressure exerted by medical staff in favour of breast-feeding. Infant formula food companies have mounted very successful advertising campaigns in Central America which have convinced women of the superiority of bottle-feeding. In Central America the bigger the baby, the better, and mothers believe that babies grow faster on the formulas. Having the tables turned so emphatically is confusing and causes distrust, so that the women do not know who to believe. Lots of encouragement and explanation will help.

Both male and female babies are loved and wanted, with no real preference for either. Sick infants will be the object of great concern. Sometimes deformity in a baby will be attributed to wrongdoing by the mother during pregnancy such as attempted abortion, excessive emotion or an unsatisfied food craving.

CHILDHOOD HEALTH AND ILLNESS

Poverty is the root cause of many of the diseases common to Central American children living in Canada. Lack of money can lead to crowded living conditions and diets deficient in fresh fruits, vegetables, and protein. This in turn encourages the spread of scabies, colds, fevers, bronchitis, and eczema. Parents use over-the-counter products to treat their children at home, but will readily bring them to see a doctor. The exception is new refugee claimants who have no medical coverage apart from the complicated bureaucratic emergency procedures provided by the Department of Immigration and Employment. Vicks VapoRub is used extensively to treat sickness in children (and adults), and a feverish baby may be completely covered with Vicks to help it fight the infection. Since bathing is thought to chill people, sick children will generally go unbathed. Swallowing a scrap of paper is believed to cause constipation in children, and parents may want to obtain a laxative.

Overall, people are receptive to vaccination. Many will be familiar with it from public health campaigns in the urban barrios of Central America, although they may not have been vaccinated themselves. Resistance may be due to a fatalistic belief that it is against God's will to prevent illness if He has determined that someone should suffer. Alternatively, people may fear that the vaccine causes infertility, a concern deriving from bad experiences with birth control campaigns or experimental drug tests in parts of the Third World.

Children, like adults, sometimes suffer the consequences of having lived in countries filled with violence. Sleep disorders, such as insomnia or nightmares which hark back to violent acts, including murders which the child has witnessed, in front of his home, sometimes occur.

CHRONIC DISEASES

Parasites and worms are chronic problems in Central America, although these can be treated and eliminated in Canada. An occasional case of active tuberculosis is found and X-rays show evidence of many more inactive cases. Malnourishment can also be an ongoing problem, and is exacerbated by the poor condition of some arriving refugee claimants and their lack of money during the first months here.

DEATH AND DYING

Because Central American countries do not generally have social programs, people look after dying members of the family themselves. If a condition is stable, the person will be taken home from the hospital to die. In urban areas, after a death occurs the body is taken to a funeral chapel where it is prepared for burial. A wake for family, close friends, and sometimes a priest is organized, usually in the presence of the open casket, and people generally stay up all night with the body. For both religious and secular people, this is very important, as it is the last time the family will be together with the deceased. Burial is the norm, cremation being a foreign idea. Catholics and Protestants will follow their customary rituals.

The mourning period traditionally requires that close family members wear black for a year. If a child dies, white clothes will be worn and for a shorter time, although both practices have become less common in recent years. A stillborn baby of religious parents will be baptized and given a burial service. Autopsies are disliked as it seems unnecessary to cut open a person who is already dead.

NUTRITION, FOOD, AND DRINK

Central American people enjoy the traditional foods of the region, such as tortillas, bean dishes, and rice seasoned with peppers and strong spices. The financial status of the family determines how much meat is eaten, with poorer working class people perhaps having meat only for Sunday dinner. Immigrants to Canada find local meat prices very high.

Breakfast is generally a substantial meal shared by the whole family, and consists of eggs, beans, and tortillas. Lunch will be eaten by family members in different locations, and may include rice, beans, or plantain as its major ingredient. Supper is a lighter family meal, perhaps of mixed vegetables. Dairy products are popular, although there is some lactose intolerance in this group. On coming to Canada, people continue to make their own tortillas at home, often buying supplies from East Indian shops where prices are the most competitive. Teenagers in North America often eat more processed and fast foods. Overall, dietary quality is seemingly high, but financial constraints make quantity a problem. Poverty also encourages diets high in carbohydrates, with resultant weight gain.

Alcohol abuse has not been noticeable among Central Americans in Canada, although there are two Spanish chapters of Alcoholics Anonymous in Vancouver. Refugee claimants overall are highly motivated to prosper in Canada and alcohol is seen as a troublesome distraction. It is sometimes used on social occasions such as after soccer games, but usually only by men. Tobacco is also not commonly used, partly because it is very expensive in Canada relative to Central America.

DENTAL PRACTICES

Except for the very small minority of wealthy immigrants, the dental status of refugee claimants is uniformly poor. Cavities, periodontal disease, and missing teeth are very common. Poverty and the absence of public health education mean that dental hygiene is unknown territory to most Central Americans. The custom has been to pull a painful tooth rather than undertake restorative work. Once in Canada, people are receptive to preventive techniques, although cost considerations will push visits to the dentist far down the list of priorities.

BATHING

People coming from poor urban barrios may have had access to water only from a single tap situated a few blocks away. The abundance of domestic running water in North America, although a relatively minor novelty, will elicit new standards of cleanliness and hygiene.

Sometimes menstruating women will not want to bathe, or wash their hair for fear of stopping the flow of menstruum. More common is the belief that people with fevers should not get wet.

CURRENT PATTERNS OF USE OF HEALTH AND SOCIAL SERVICES

The point which a person has reached in the immigration procedure greatly influences how she or he will utilize medical services. Before refugee status is granted, claimants have no medical insurance except for the federal emergency procedures, which require lengthy paperwork. These people are very conscious of their vulnerability and will wait a long time before seeking help. Alternatively, they seek free services such as the Pine Free Clinic in Vancouver. Refugees who have been accepted and who qualify for provincial health insurance often make frequent initial visits to the doctor and for apparently minor problems. But as they adjust to the community and their lives become less stressful, these visits drop off. People will also use emergency services as necessary. Once they accept the notion of a long-term family physician, they may try to find a Spanish-speaking doctor. Alternatively, they use a volunteer translator to accompany them.

Social programs have a mixed reception. Welfare is demoralizing and can increase stress levels. Other services, such as counselling or family resources, are underutilized because of the lack of available Spanish speakers and the natural Latin reserve about discussing private matters with strangers. Because these people have endured political and psychological violence, the need for adequate counselling facilities is self-evident.

POLITICAL VIOLENCE AND TORTURE

Physicians examining refugee claimants frequently come across evidence of torture and brutality. The natural temptation is to confront the patient, albeit with compassion, and seek explanations. But this may be a grave error which will only occasion distress in victims of this type of violence. The pain goes far deeper than physical wounds, and a lengthy period, perhaps two or three years, is needed before professional and patient develop the necessary degree of trust.

The legacy of civil war and politically sponsored abduction, murder, and torture will also often show up in people's sleep. Children are haunted by nightmares, adults are plagued by sleeplessness, and families mourn those who have been killed, imprisoned, or caused to "disappear." Although not everyone has been a victim, everybody knows a friend or family member who has suffered. For the Canadian health professional, it is very important to take account of this background—but to wait until the patient raises the subject.

DELIVERING CULTURALLY SENSITIVE HEALTH CARE

The old adage about putting yourself in someone else's shoes is perhaps the best advice for providing compassionate and appropriate health care to immigrants from Central America. Uncovering the details of a patient's story will help in building this understanding. Country of origin, social background, current immigration status, and length of intermediate stay in the U.S. all help to reveal the situation left behind, language skills, familiarity with North American customs, and the legal status of individual immigrant patients. Refugees are in a very stressful position and need social as well as medical support. On the other hand, it is essential to guard against being patronizing. Poverty and limited English do not preclude pride and mental alertness. As one physician put it, "People are more fragile because of what they have been through. They really don't want to be bothersome, they don't want to make waves. So a doctor will have to take time and be gentle, but the rewards will be great."

Another Vancouver physician has prepared a mimeographed sheet in Spanish which explains how the medical system works, what a call schedule is, and what to do in case of emergency. For people with limited skills in English, instructions should be very clear and direct, such as "See your family doctor tomorrow," or "Come back in one week." Hospital forms will need translation. People should be told clearly that they have a right to ask for help and care. And health professionals should not mistake apparent passivity for acceptance. In fact, it may be a simple case of the patient not understanding the English expressions being used.

FURTHER READING

Acker, Alison. *Children of the Volcano*. Toronto: Between the Lines Press 1986

Cabezas, Orar. *Fire from the Mountain: The Making of a Sandinista*. New York, NY: Crown 1985

Calvert, Peter. *Guatemala: A Nation in Turmoil*. Boulder, CO: Westview Press 1985

Cohn, Jorgen, et al. "Torture of Children: An Investigation of Chilean Immigrant Children in Denmark, Preliminary Report," *Child Abuse and Neglect*, Vol. 5 (1981): 201-3

Cosminsky, S. "Childbirth and Change: A Guatemalan Study," in *Ethnography of Fertility and Birth*, ed. Carol MacCormack. New York, NY: Academic Press 1982

Ferris, Elizabeth G. "Regional Responses to Central American Refugees: Policy Making in Nicaragua, Honduras, and Mexico," in *Refugees and World Politics*, ed. E. Ferris. New York, NY: Praeger 1985

Menchu, Rigoberta. *I, Rigoberta Menchu: An Indian Woman in Guatemala*. London: Verso 1984

Maduro, Renaldo. "Curanderismo and Latino Views of Disease and Curing," *The Western Journal of Medicine*, Vol. 139, No. 6 (1983): 64-70

Randall, Margaret. *Sandino's Daughters*. Vancouver, BC: New Star Books 1981

CONTRIBUTORS

Augusto Arana (Immigrant Services Society, Vancouver)
Roxana Aune (MOSAIC, Vancouver)
Gill Bentzen (Immigrant Services Society, Vancouver)

Bernardo Berdichewsky (Capilano College, North Vancouver)
Althea Brown (Vancouver Health Department, Burrard Unit)
Yaya de Andrade (VAST, Vancouver)
Esther Frid (Family Services, Vancouver)
Miriam Maurer (MOSAIC, Vancouver)
Carolina Palacios (Vancouver)
Peter Quelch (Richmond)
Sheila Shannon (MOSAIC, Vancouver)
Lucia Silva-Zarate (Inland Refugee Society, Vancouver)

CHAPTER FOUR

The Chinese

Magdalene C. Lai and Ka-Ming Kevin Yue

INTRODUCTION

The Chinese ethnic group in Canada is composed of people from a variety of regions. The ancestors of the majority of these Chinese originated in mainland China, Hong Kong, and Taiwan. However, Chinese continue to emigrate from other Southeast Asian countries including Singapore, Thailand, Malaysia, Vietnam, Cambodia, and Laos. A large number of Chinese residing in Canada also originated in other parts of the world such as Fiji, Africa, and the West Indies. This chapter will concentrate on the Chinese from mainland China, Hong Kong, and Taiwan, as they represent the largest proportion of immigrants to Canada. However, the ethnic Chinese from other countries have much in common with them.

GEOGRAPHY AND HISTORY

People's Republic of China

After Russia and Canada, China is the third largest country in the world with the world's largest population. China's vast land area includes deserts, mountains, and farmland and its climate ranges from severe desert conditions, long cold winters in Tibet and northern Manchuria, to tropical warmth and rain in the coastal areas of the southeast.

Most of its population resides in the eastern third of the country where the major cities and fertile plains are located. About 80 per cent of the population live in rural villages. Agriculture is the backbone of China's economy although industry is rapidly expanding.

About 94 per cent of the population is Han, which has been the largest national group in China for centuries. The Han share a common history, culture, and written language, although dialects vary from region to region. The rest of the population is composed of about fifty minority groups, most of whom live in the border regions of the far north and west.

The Chinese view their country as "the centre of the world." It has a rich culture that developed during the course of many successive empires which date back as early as 3,500 years. In 221 BC a strong, centralized Chinese empire was established and lasted in some form or other for a period of 2,000 years. During the 1800s, the empire started to weaken and it was overthrown by revolutionaries in 1911. In 1912, China became a republic ruled by the Nationalist party. After much turmoil, the Chinese Communist party defeated the Nationalists in 1949, and set up the present government. The state's official name was changed to the People's Republic of China.

Under communist rule, all important industries, trade, and finance were placed under state ownership and direction. Where land was owned and farmed by individual families in the past, its management was now turned over to large community groups. People dissatisfied with communist domination fled to neighbouring states or applied to Western countries for refugee status.

After years of political hardship and turmoil, the government not only dramatically increased industrial production, but also expanded and improved education and medical care. The latter is completely socialized. Professional government workers are provided free medical insurance, and insurance fees for the other workers, mostly farmers, are deducted from their wages (Wong 1987).

The recent recognition of the People's Republic of China by Western countries, and China's desire to promote technological advance by opening its doors to the Western world, have led to further changes in the lives of the Chinese. Moreover, the Chinese government's recent emphasis on private ownership signifies further economic changes to come.

Hong Kong

Situated on the coast of China, Hong Kong's 410 square miles include Hong Kong island, a peninsula attached to mainland China, and more than 235 islets. Hong Kong has a subtropical climate with hot and humid summers and occasional typhoons, and winters that are dry and cool.

Hong Kong is one of the most densely populated places in the world. Because of its strategic location and its status as a free port, it is a bustling centre of economic activity, with one of the strongest and most varied economies in Asia. The vital importance of international trade, finance, and tourism means that the majority of residents, men and women, work for manufacturing firms or have jobs in commerce. Less than 3 per cent make their living by farming or fishing.

Almost all—approximately 98 per cent—the residents of Hong Kong are Chinese. In the past, large numbers of people have migrated from China to seek employment and, more recently, to escape communist rule in China. The two official languages in Hong Kong are Chinese and English, Cantonese being the most commonly used dialect.

Until the 1800s, Hong Kong was part of China and consisted of a few small fishing and farming villages. After the Opium War of 1839 between China and Great Britain, the island of Hong Kong became a British colony. Following further disputes between the two countries, Britain gained control of Kowloon peninsula in 1860. In 1898, China leased the New Territories to Britain for ninety-nine years. The government of China claims that Hong Kong still belongs to China and, as a result of an agreement with Britain, plans to repossess the colony in 1997.

In the past, large numbers of Chinese from Hong Kong have emigrated to Canada and the United States. Currently the unpredictable political future of Hong Kong is creating much anxiety; some people fear that strict communist domination will be implanted after 1997. This uncertainty has led large numbers of Chinese, mostly from the higher socio-economic classes, to resettle in countries such as Canada, the United States, and Australia.

Taiwan

Taiwan is a mountainous island in the South China Sea situated about ninety miles off the Chinese coast. It has a subtropical climate with hot, humid summers and mild winters.

Most Taiwanese are Chinese whose ancestors originated in the Fukien and Kwangtung provinces of mainland China. Although the people speak various Chinese dialects, depending on their regional birthplaces, almost all speak Mandarin, the official Chinese language. About one-third of the population are farmers, whereas a majority is involved in manufacturing and foreign trade.

The Chinese of Taiwan came to the island from mainland China as early as the sixth century AD but large-scale settlement did not begin until about 1600. In 1895, Japan gained control of Taiwan as a result of the First Sino-Japanese War and developed and expanded Taiwan's agriculture, industry, and transportation networks. China regained Taiwan after the Second World War.

In 1949, when the Chinese communists took control of mainland China, the defeated nationalist government under Chiang Kai-Shek settled in Taiwan. Both the communist and the nationalist governments consider Taiwan a province of China, but each claims to be the legal ruler of all of China. In the 1970s, a number of nations, including the United States, cut diplomatic relations with Taiwan and established ties with Communist China.

MIGRATION TO CANADA

There are many reasons why Chinese have come to Canada. Some want to live in a modern and agreeable society, while others feel that Canada offers better job opportunities for them and better educational facilities for their children. Many come to join the relatives who have already settled here. Still others from China, and now Hong Kong, wish to escape from communist rule and prefer living in a democratic society.

The greatest influx of Chinese was between 1881 and 1884, when over 15,000 men were "imported" from China to serve as construction workers on the Canadian Pacific Railway. In 1923, with the passing of the Exclusion Act, the entry of Chinese into Canada virtually ceased (Starkins 1986). Immigration increased slightly after the Second World War when Canada allowed close relatives of Chinese residents to enter the country (Statistics Canada 1981a).

The repeal of the discriminatory clauses of Canadian immigration laws in 1962, and the development of the "point system" encouraged a large number of Chinese to emigrate to Canada, especially after the Hong Kong riots in 1967 (Statistics Canada 1981b).

By 1978, a new Immigration Act had come into force and marked a turning point in Chinese immigration; the point system was revised to emphasize occupational experience and demand. With this new policy, Chinese immigrants, especially those who could generate employment in Canada, were encouraged to settle. As a result between 1978 and 1981, Asians accounted for 43.8 per cent of all immigrants to Canada (Statistics Canada 1981b). Hong Kong Chinese with relatives resident in Canada, or who were skilled workers and professionals began to arrive. Canada also opened its doors to a large number of Southeast Asian refugees from mainland China and Vietnam (Statistics Canada 1981b). In the face of China's imminent take-over of Hong Kong in 1997, more people from the colony with investment capital or the capacity to create employment have moved to Canada, as have a number of retired people (Employment and Immigration Canada 1985).

The majority of Chinese immigrants have moved to urban areas like Vancouver or Toronto. The mild weather in western Canada makes it particularly attractive to these immigrants who are used to a tropical climate. Some feel more at ease living on the west coast because their home country is only "on the other side of the Pacific Ocean."

SOCIO-ECONOMIC STATUS

Socio-economic status among immigrants varies from well-to-do families who bring their lifelong savings to invest in Canada, to low income refugees who have to work long hours to support their families. Educational background also ranges from professionals who are university educated to people with no education who are illiterate in both English and their home language.

Often, due to lack of English or different skill demands in Canada, immigrants experience downward occupational mobility, or worse, unemployment. For example, it is not surprising to find a doctor schooled in Chinese medicine who works long hours as a restaurant helper in Canada. Many immigrants value employment highly, and consider it to be the equivalent of the "rice bowl." Dissatisfaction with employment status often contributes to stress.

EXPERIENCE WITH CANADIANS

According to Anthony Chan (1983) in *Gold Mountain*, "racism is woven into Canada's evolution" (p. 15). The Chinese who were early immigrants experienced extreme hardship and racial discrimination. It is only in the last few decades that they have been more widely accepted as part of Canada's multicultural society.

Many immigrants, especially the younger generation, often adapt well. They are reputed to be hard-working individuals who make little trouble and conform to the rules of society. With some exceptions, experiences of rejection and prejudice have been infrequently voiced by Chinese in recent years.

RELIGION

Traditionally, many people from China are Buddhists. In Canada there are often Buddhist temples in large cities, and small shrines may be placed in homes and in restaurants as tokens of respect for the gods and ancestors. In addition, incense is burned and offerings are made on special feast days. Some Chinese believe strongly that one's past lives influence one's present and future lives; for example evil deeds from a past life cause serious illness in the present and threaten the future.

Roman Catholic and Protestant Chinese have founded churches in Canada which not only provide religious support but also opportunities for socialization, help in finding jobs, counselling, day care centres, and Chinese classes.

FESTIVALS AND RELIGIOUS HOLIDAYS

Special events and holidays are celebrated as feast days, when families gather for meals together. Major Chinese festivals include Chinese New Year, the mid-Autumn Festival, and the Dragon Festival. Often, the Chinese in Canada celebrate both Chinese and Canadian festivals.

LANGUAGE

Early immigrants from China mainly spoke the Taosan dialect. More recent arrivals from China, Hong Kong, and Taiwan speak different dialects of Chinese depending on the region in which they were born. In general though, most people from Taiwan and northern China speak Mandarin and most southern and Hong Kong Chinese speak Cantonese. Many people from China do not speak English whereas those from Hong Kong and Taiwan have often learned English in school.

In Canada, attendance at English classes may be difficult for those who have little access to transport or who work ten to twelve hours a day. It is also particularly difficult for restaurant workers who are often occupied in the evenings.

FAMILY STRUCTURE

The traditional Chinese family is often large, extended, lives together, and is headed by the eldest working male. A single household may include parents, children, children's spouses, and grandchildren. Unmarried children live at home until marriage, but some may leave later.

Traditionally, the Chinese take pride in having large families. The greater the number of people and generations there are together, the better. The family is so important that the Chinese have specific terms for each member. Instead of a person being merely an "uncle," he may be addressed as "the second eldest brother of one's mother." Traditionally, the elderly are highly respected and the young are obliged to take care of them.

In the past, it was the husband who interacted with the outside world. To some extent this still obtains. He works, takes care of finances, and usually disciplines the children. He also makes the primary family decisions. The wife, on the other hand, runs the household and cares for the children. She is usually responsible for routine health decisions. For example, she decides on the choice of birth control, in consultation with her husband. Serious decision-making may involve husband, wife, *and* extended family. Health professionals therefore need to be alert to family decision-making patterns. Communication with all members concerned may be necessary in any given situation.

In Canada, family members may be physically separated because some are not eligible for immigration or for reasons of work. Immigrants often work extremely hard to send money back home to family members.

Sometimes the husband, due to a poor command of English, may depend on his children to communicate with outsiders, and this may be degrading for him. On the other hand, the wife is often forced to work as well as look after her family, leaving her with the feeling that she is doing both jobs inadequately. She may also be faced with conflicting expectations: Western liberated woman on the one hand versus traditional housewife on the other. Conflicts may also arise between the daughter-in-law and the mother-in-law, due to contrasting lifestyles and values.

Generational conflicts are compounded when parents only speak Chinese while their children learn English and gradually forget their native language. Severe communication barriers may result, with parents and children hardly talking to each other.

Families may also experience conflicts because of numerous other factors. Frustrations may arise when families find difficulty in living in a foreign country, and in adapting to a new lifestyle and environment. Expectations of the new country may also go unfulfilled. For example, the husband expecting to provide his family with a comfortable life in Canada may be unable to find a job. His wife becomes the bread-winner while he is forced to adopt a "woman's role." In addition, a Chinese couple's relationship may deteriorate if they are not used to discussing their problems with each other. Potential difficulties arise when the Chinese put more energy into meeting the family's physical requirements than into communicating with each other.

CHILD-REARING

Traditionally, the birth of a male child is considered more desirable than the birth of a female, since the male carries the family name and is entitled to a larger family inheritance. Male children are especially desired in China where, at times, a one child policy has been enforced. In the old days, if a wife was "unable" to bear a male child, the husband often took a second wife.

Parenting and early education traditionally take place within the home. Babies are breast-fed or formula-fed. In the past the rich hired "wet nurses" to breast-feed their babies. Rice soon becomes the infant's staple food. Toilet-training is initiated at an early age. Babies are generally bathed more often than in the West and, from the Western point of view, parents often overdress their children to prevent them from catching colds. Discipline may appear harsh to the Westerner and open gestures of affection are seldom displayed. Parents may feel that their primary responsibility to their children is to fulfil their material needs, that is, to ensure that they are properly fed and clothed.

In Canada the poor family may send the children to work as they grow up, or to serve apprenticeships, and the rich family usually sends them to university. Work and education are highly valued and are seen as the only means of climbing the social ladder. Expending time on jobs and schooling is considered much more important than leisure activities. Personal success is often measured in terms of level of education and the amount of money earned to support the family.

Difficulties arise when children do not meet their parents' high expectations of them at school. This sometimes triggers serious mental health problems in children. The increased frustrations experienced by parents may cause physical abuse of children or wives.

As some parents lack a good command of English, the oldest child who speaks English may be given a great deal of family responsibility, almost acquiring the role of parent.

MARRIAGE PATTERNS

The traditional Chinese marriage is arranged jointly by a match-maker and the parents according to their social status, wealth, and their ancestors' place of birth. A dowry from the bride's family may consist of a roasted suckling pig and pastries, while the groom's family may present furnishings for the couple's new home. Divorces are rare. Traditionally, the wife is expected to yield to and tolerate the husband's wishes. In Canada, however, individual choice of marriage partner is preferred, so that most couples are not matched in the traditional manner. Interracial marriage exists but is frequently frowned upon by the elderly. Divorce rates in Canada are also on the rise.

THE ELDERLY

A large number of elderly Chinese reside in Canada. The surviving pioneers who migrated to Canada in the late 1800s and early 1900s have now reached an advanced age. Most were unable or unwilling to return home after they came to Canada but settled instead in various cities in British Columbia. Legislation passed between 1885 and 1923 prevented the families of these men from joining them. As a result they formed clan associations to provide each other with support and care as they age and approach death (Starkins 1986).

A second group of elderly Chinese have come more recently to join their families. After they arrive in Canada they often inherit household and child care duties because their children go out to work to support the family. Their daily duties, together with their lack of English, sometimes prevent them from getting out and feelings of isolation often result. If they live in a large city their only outlet may be a bus trip to the local Chinatown where they can meet people speaking a familiar language.

Another group of elderly are the well-to-do Chinese who have chosen to spend their retirement years in Canada. Many are not familiar with the health care system and are unaware of resources available to them.

Generational conflicts may occur between adult children and elderly parents especially where they have immigrated at different times and have been separated for long periods. As a result, older family members and younger children may have difficulty in adjusting to each other's lifestyles. In addition, parents often bring with them the culture, values, and beliefs of their native lands, whereas their children may have adapted to the Western way of living.

CULTURAL VALUES AND BEHAVIOUR

The Chinese name usually consists of a one-word surname followed by a two-word given name. Some families, notably those ones from

South Africa, had their names reversed by immigration authorities. A woman may keep her own surname or use her own and her husband's surnames in hyphenated form. The more traditional Chinese may give a child a second name when schooling commences and a third name when marriage occurs. In Canada, the child may have an additional English name.

People usually greet one another by bowing their heads and smiling. Indirect eye contact may be a sign of respect. Body contact beyond a hand shake, for example, kissing and hugging, is uncommon and is usually avoided with strangers. To the Westerner's eyes, the polite and formal Chinese may appear reserved and unassertive.

When dealing with conflicts, the Chinese may traditionally be persuaded by others without asserting their own rights. They may prefer to listen to what others have to say instead of confronting them directly. And they may nod and smile when they neither understand nor agree with what is being said. They may then reply in an indirect way and try to handle the situation diplomatically. Generally, they respect authority, abide by the law, and heed the wishes of the elderly.

Chinese are generally pragmatic people. Priority is given to satisfying practical family needs, particularly for sufficient food and clothing. It may then be hard for parents to understand why further demands are made on them, for example, to meet a child's emotional needs.

An invitation is required to visit another home, but hospitality is very important. Typically, the Chinese like to be surrounded by many relatives and friends; the more people there are, the better. When a person is hospitalized, family members may prefer to visit as a group.

Some Chinese may not be familiar with the need to make appointments with health professionals and sometimes appointments may be missed through work obligations.

TRADITIONAL CONCEPTS OF HEALTH AND ILLNESS

The Chinese concept of health and illness is based on Chinese medicine which is divided into three distinct but related types: classical Chinese medicine, Chinese folk medicine, and medicine in contemporary China (Gould-Martin and Ngin 1981).

Classical Chinese medicine is recorded in ancient texts: *Huang Ti Nei Ching (The Yellow Emperor's Classic of Internal Medicine)*, believed to have been written between 2698 and 2598 BC; the *Shang Han Lun*

(Treatise on Fevers); and the *Shen Nung Pen Ts'ao Ching (Shen Nung's Classic Pharmacopoeia)*—the last two written around the third century BC.

According to the *Nei Ching*, man is inseparable from his universe, which is viewed as a vast, indivisible entity. All of man and nature are related to each other in a harmonious balance. Individuals must adjust themselves wholly to the environment and maintain this balance, since imbalance brings illness. Five elements—wood, fire, earth, metal, and water—form the universe.

The *Nei Ching* especially emphasized the concepts of yin and yang, which permeate all of nature. Health is a state of spiritual and physical harmony with nature, in which yin and yang are in dynamic equilibrium. Illness, on the other hand, represents an imbalance or disequilibrium in these forces.

The concept of yin and yang originated in the southern provinces of China. The majority of people who live in China, Hong Kong, or Taiwan originally came from southern China, and have strong beliefs in these concepts.

Various parts of the human body correspond to the dualistic principles of yin and yang. Yang also represents the positive, male energy that produces light, warmth, and fullness. Yin represents the female, negative energy, the force of darkness, coldness, and emptiness (Spector 1979). The human body is viewed as a gift from parents and forebears, and should be well cared for and preserved.

Chinese folk medicine bases many of its ideas on classical sources, but the concepts may hold different meanings. "Hot" and "cold" are often substituted for yang and yin, although harmonious balance must be maintained between the two opposing forces. People often rely on information about treatment obtained from newspapers, by word of mouth, and from traditions passed on down the generations, without fully understanding how the treatment works. Religion and magic may also enter into folk medicine. The Chinese may attribute health to good luck or to leading a good life, either in the past or the present. They may consult doctors knowledgeable about Chinese folk medicine who prescribe herbal teas for specific ailments.

Chinese medicine in contemporary China draws ideas from classical and folk traditions and from current medical advances, both Chinese and Western. Medical treatment from either broad tradition, or both, may be offered to cure illnesses. If the Chinese in Canada find treatment unsuccessful here, it is not uncommon for them to return to their homeland to seek help from specialists in Chinese medicine.

HEALTH CARE FACILITIES IN CHINA, HONG KONG, AND TAIWAN

In China, medical insurance is offered to two groups of people. Public workers (office workers, civil servants, and professionals) who are employed primarily by the government get free medical insurance. Farmers have the medical insurance premiums deducted from their wages (Wong 1987).

Patients, for the most part, seek health care through clinics set up in the farm communes or factories. From there, patients may be referred to district hospitals and, if necessary, to city hospitals, then finally to university hospitals if more specialized treatment is necessary. When patients go to hospitals they do not necessarily see the same doctor each time (Wong 1987).

In China, most doctors have some training in both Western and Chinese medicine, and most facilities employ both types of physician in varying proportions. Thus health care is mostly a combination of both Western and Chinese medicine. For example, surgery may be performed along Western lines while anaesthesia may be administered by acupuncture (Wong 1987). The forms of treatment offered by Chinese medicine include herbal medicine, acupuncture, acupressure (application of pressure to certain points on the body), moxibustion (the burning of small quantities of dried herbs on the body), and chiropractic bone setting. When patients seek help from hospitals, they may encounter specialists and not general practitioners. This contrasts with the Canadian system where the general practitioner is usually responsible for the overall care of the patient.

There are basically two systems of care in Hong Kong. One system includes private doctors and specialists. Clients using this system are usually well off people who rely heavily on social contacts to see the "best" specialist. Others who cannot afford the high fees usually use the second system, the government out-patient clinics. As these clinics may have over 100 patients per day, they are extremely overcrowded and people often have to line up for hours. Usually they see a different doctor each time and the physician's interviews may be brief.

Likewise there are two types of hospital in Hong Kong: expensive private hospitals where patients may have private rooms and bring their private nurses, and government hospitals used by the poor. In the latter, large proportions of staff are people in training. Although these hospitals offer advanced and specialized treatment, they cannot accommodate large numbers of patients. An additional system of care is provided by unlicensed doctors who may have had training in Chinese or Western medicine but never qualified.

The system of medicine in Taiwan includes government-sponsored health services, private physicians and hospitals, and physicians who practise traditional Chinese medicine. The private health services are more expensive and thus cater to the more affluent (Kleinman 1980).

In most of the countries from which the Chinese have moved there are also a variety of practitioners of folk medicine, such as herbalists, shamans, fortune tellers, and priests who offer services to sick people.

As Chinese people are extremely diverse they may have very different preferences in health care. In mainland China, people may not see Western doctors frequently and they often medicate themselves or use Chinese doctors. In Vietnam, some use Chinese medicine exclusively. However, in Hong Kong most people go to both Chinese and Western doctors.

ATTITUDES TO ILLNESS

Illness may be seen as a loss of balance in yin and yang, or an imbalance in hot and cold foods. Causes of illness may include foods that are excessively hot or cold, but also foods that are believed to be "poisonous." Germs, fate, and bad luck are also held to cause disease. For example, a young man may apparently develop flu, with fever and chills, but will attribute his illness to having eaten a roast duck, which he perceives as poisonous. Similarly, a pregnant woman usually avoids poisonous foods such as shellfish or mutton. Parents of children with asthma or chronic coughs may refuse them cold drinks like iced water, or fruits and vegetables because their illness is thought to be caused by excessive cold.

People usually think of themselves as ill only when symptoms are evident. Their primary goal is then to get rid of the symptoms. They may have difficulty understanding the implications of chronic illnesses where symptoms persist for a long time and there is no absolute cure.

In Chinese medicine, people may seek cures from substances which they associate with their own deficiency. For instance, a traditional Chinese may eat animals' brains in order to grow wiser. A diabetic may eat an animals' pancreas in the hope of cure. People thought to be anaemic often eat red foods. These examples illustrate why traditional Chinese may have difficulty in regarding plastic capsules as a cure.

ATTITUDE TOWARDS WESTERN AND CHINESE MEDICINE

According to many Chinese acute illnesses and those requiring surgery, for example, appendicitis and gallstones, are best treated by Western medicine. Chinese medicine is usually used to treat conditions with prolonged symptoms, like chronic colds, coughs, internal disorders such as ulcers, and chronic illnesses like diabetes, hypertension, pneumonia, and asthma. When serious relapses occur, the Chinese may revert to Western doctors.

PREVALENCE OF DISEASES

Certain diseases are more prevalent in the Chinese population than others: hepatitis, tuberculosis, intestinal parasites, and renal stones. Some types of cancer are also more prevalent in Chinese groups including nasopharyngeal cancer, esophageal cancer, liver cancer, and gastric cancer. Many Chinese are intolerant of lactose and cannot easily digest milk or milk products.

MENTAL HEALTH

The Chinese are more likely to explain the causes of mental illness in terms of external factors or events and the problem is usually presented in the form of somatic complaints. For example, an elderly lady may say that her heart hurts and may go to the coronary care unit for help when she is actually suffering from depression. Traditionally, different emotions are perceived to be closely related to different organs. For example, anger is associated with the liver, and joy and depression with the heart (Li 1987). Consequently, clients may seek relief of physical symptoms but not discuss mental health problems. Patients may also attribute their illnesses to supernatural forces like evil spirits, or excessively cold winds. They may not understand the therapies used in Canada; talking about problems may not be an acceptable form of treatment.

Family members have a great influence on how mental health is viewed. Some families may be overprotective of, and give refuge to, their mentally ill members and the illness becomes a family secret. They may also refuse treatment because they view mental illness as bringing shame on the family. Families may also fear that the mental health problems are genetically inherited. Consequently, people who do have mental health problems may be reluctant to seek help and may delay doing so (Lee 1986).

Health professionals must find ways to ensure that clients have access to good care but they must also try to be patient so as to win the family's trust. Reassurances about strict confidentiality may comfort family members, as might genetic counselling to clients whose families believe that mental health problems are inherited (Lee 1986).

RELATIONSHIP BETWEEN PATIENT AND PROFESSIONAL

Chinese patients and health professionals often come from varied locations, different socio-economic classes, and diverse cultures. In particular, Chinese professionals who work in Canada are likely to be Canadian- or Hong Kong-born and may be of a higher socio-economic class than their patients. For these reasons Chinese professionals and patients may not always share the same health beliefs.

Chinese patients often bring experiences from their home country to their encounters with professionals in Canada. For example, in China patients usually request their preferred treatments from their doctors. These same patients may appear rude and aggressive in Canada when they behave in this way.

The concept of preventive medicine may be unfamiliar to some Chinese who only will seek help when they feel ill. They may be unfamiliar with annual check-ups and the continual monitoring of their health. Also, Chinese patients may not have experience of detailed medical histories or understand the need for them.

In their home countries Chinese patients have generally been taught to respect doctors and not to ask questions. Health professionals in Canada must therefore ensure that patients adequately understand the diagnosis, treatment, and necessary medical procedures.

In Canada, the language barrier remains a considerable obstacle for many patients. Most often, patients are limited to the small number of health care workers who speak their language. Even though it is not always appropriate, children or Chinese-speaking workers are sometimes asked to interpret.

Chinese women may prefer female professionals, especially for obstetric and gynaecological care. Similarly, Chinese males may be unfamiliar with the idea of seeing female professionals.

Patients may prefer older more experienced health professionals. They may also have very high expectations of medical treatment; thus it is crucial to explain to Chinese patients the real limits of the treatment in order to avoid misunderstanding and disappointment.

Due to language barriers and their lack of general resources, the Chinese may feel the need to have a close relationship with professionals. They may ask professionals to be friends and call on them for non-medical help.

For Chinese who are used to one or two main health practitioners in their home country, the Western health care system with its team approach may appear confusing. Nursing is not highly regarded as a profession in their home countries. However, community health nurses or professionals entrusted with specific tasks, such as prenatal classes or teaching home management of diabetes, may be well respected because patients can discern their specific responsibilities. However, Chinese often confuse these professionals with physicians whom they see as the primary health care givers.

HOSPITALIZATION

Hospitalized patients may encounter both language and cultural barriers. For example, in their home countries family members and friends are expected to visit ill patients in a group, yet in Canada they discover that hospital policy discourages this. At home, family members may also be ready and willing to help in nursing the hospitalized person, especially elderly patients. Consequently Chinese families are often confused by Canadian hospital policies.

Since elderly Chinese often associate hospitalization with death they may prove reluctant hospital patients. On the other hand, family members may rush an elderly parent to the hospital, thinking that he or she may receive better treatment for the illness.

The death of a person at home is considered to bring bad luck.

MEDICATION AND TREATMENT

Self-medication is a common practice. Ill Chinese patients may take both Western and Chinese medicine, plus home cures, particularly oils and ointments.

Chinese want immediate results from medications, especially as only one or two doses of Chinese medicine are needed to relieve symptoms. Therefore, they may question prolonged Western treatment regimes. For example, they may prematurely discontinue taking an antibiotic prescribed for two weeks since they do not detect immediate results.

Chinese believe in "all things in moderation." Thus taking medicine over an extended period of time may be felt to weaken their bodies (Li 1987). Often they feel that Western medicine is too potent for them or their small bodies and they may reduce dosages to a quantity they believe suitable. For example, an elderly Chinese with diabetes may reduc his insulin because it is "foreign" and jeopardizes his health. It is crucial for health professionals to give patients specific and clear instructions about medications.

Injections are often regarded as more effective than pills, and pills in turn are considered more effective than drops.

Chinese clients often emphasize that medicine must be compatible with their bodies and this is indicated by the resultant degree of symptomatic relief. Clients may also associate symptomatic relief with the doctor's skill rather than the effectiveness of the medicine. It is not uncommon for patients to attribute cures to the doctor, not the medicine.

Chinese may refuse blood tests as they believe loss of blood will weaken their bodies or that these tests are too invasive.

The Chinese value the wholeness of the body and thus they may avoid surgery because it is a form of mutilation; surgery is resorted to only if all other treatments fail. For example, parents may refuse corrective surgery for a child with a congenital heart defect if the child does not display obvious symptoms of illness. They may also not accept the need for, and thus will delay, cosmetic surgery to correct conditions like dislocated hips or strabismus.

REHABILITATION

Rehabilitation services for family members who are physically or mentally handicapped may be avoided. For example, parents may refuse exercises for a child with muscle weakness because they view physiotherapy as painful to the child.

Chinese parents of mentally handicapped children may prefer to accept the child's present condition rather than use rehabilitation services or they may refuse help from outsiders because they are ashamed of the child's "abnormality." As a result, mentally handicapped children may lack life experience and exposure to the outside world.

FAMILY PLANNING

Traditional Chinese prefer large families. Male children, especially the first born are highly valued, because the family name is assured. In China, intrauterine devices and birth control pills are commonly used. Some families from China may request therapeutic abortions on the basis of their experience of the Chinese government's family planning and the single child family policies.

Some Chinese couples in Canada may be unfamiliar with family planning methods. Couples often rely on hearsay for information and women may consult relatives or friends. Knowledgeable men may choose the method while the responsibility for implementation of birth control may rest with the woman. Few women use diaphragms, because of unfamiliarity with their own bodies. Some women may request tubal ligations after they have had three or four children.

PREGNANCY AND PRENATAL CARE

The Chinese maintain certain prenatal cultural practices to safeguard the foetus in the mother's womb. Women may avoid excessively hot foods like lamb, or excessively cold foods such as watermelon and banana, or poisonous foods such as shellfish. Women may also avoid foods with a slippery texture for fear their babies may slip out.

Couples may not be able to attend prenatal classes because of work commitments, transport problems, or language difficulties.

Prenatal care in rural mainland China is sometimes not sought until very late in pregnancy. This attitude may persist in some recent Chinese immigrants.

The postpartum period is often seen as a vulnerable, cold period characterized by an excess of yin. Chinese mothers may therefore avoid cold foods like salads, bananas, fruit juices, or cold water. They also try to eat more hot foods, for example, sweet vinegars, chicken, eggs, and certain types of herbs, in an attempt to balance yin and yang. Couples may traditionally abstain from sex for 100 days after childbirth.

The current trend in mainland China is to breast-feed; immigrants from Hong Kong will probably prefer to bottle-feed.

CHILDBIRTH

In Canada, childbirth is sometimes a difficult time for a Chinese immigrant woman. She may be unable to communicate with hospital staff about her needs and may believe that procedures like epidurals are harmful and cause severe headaches and backaches.

During the perinatal period, the mother, mother-in-law, aunts, and sisters may help the pregnant woman. In recent years in Canada, Chinese husbands have participated more actively in childbirth and take time off to help with baby care. However, some Chinese husbands still feel uncomfortable about such activities.

Upon discharge from hospital, the woman may expect that her helpers, for example, her mother or a nanny, will care for her baby. Her reliance on others in no way indicates her uninterest in the child.

POSTPARTUM PERIOD

The postpartum period is considered dangerous because the woman is susceptible to excessive coldness. Often, elderly relatives warn her that if she does not take care of herself she may suffer long-term consequences such as rheumatism or enduring pain in her limbs. To relieve the cold she must avoid cold foods, and cold winds. Cold foods include most vegetables, fruits, and fruit juices. She must also stay inside to avoid cold winds; this common practice is called "sitting for the month." Cold water is avoided by not bathing or washing hair for a month, and heavy lifting is avoided to safeguard the uterus. She may not take her baby out (even to visit the doctor) for fear her child may be exposed to the cold winds.

NUTRITION AND FOOD

The central dietary tenet is the balancing of yin and yang, and cold and hot foods. People with a hot disease often balance their diet with cold foods, and vice versa. Soup is a vital home remedy, taken almost daily to maintain health and for dietary balance. Families often drink the soup extract, but not the vegetables or meat ingredients (Koo 1984).

Food has very important social meaning for families since mealtimes are the main occasion for the family to come together. Feasts occur on special occasions such as birthdays, weddings, or family births.

Milk is taken infrequently because it is disliked and because many Chinese are intolerant of lactose. Professionals may suggest substitutes such as soya milk, lactaid, tofu, or calcium substitutes. Rice is a major staple for the southern Chinese, while flour products such as noodles or dumplings, are the equivalent for the northern Chinese. Rice is considered neutral, neither hot nor cold. For many southern Chinese, rice is almost a necessity for every meal; a person has not eaten well without rice. However, some Chinese eat excessive amounts of starch or sugar in the forms of sweetbreads, buns, rice, and noodles.

Chinese try to eat two or three meals a day, but these may not always be well balanced nutritionally. Some diets consist primarily of carbohydrates like rice, congee, noodles, or bread, with little meat. School children and working adults may miss breakfast because parents have insufficient time for preparation. Adults eating irregular meals sometimes develop ulcers or gastric discomforts. Sometimes the response to these discomforts is the avoidance of further eating, in the belief that the symptoms will go away. Moreover, when people are sick, other food restrictions are imposed.

Diets may vary according to social class, with the rich eating larger quantities of meat and the poor more bread and cereals. Some preserved foods, such as ducks' eggs, fish, and vegetables, are often high in sodium as are many common condiments such as monosodium glutamate (MSG), soya and oyster sauce. (Low sodium soya sauce is available in Canada.) Some foods have a high fat content as they are prepared with lard.

Chinese males often smoke cigarettes heavily. While alcohol may be socially acceptable, some Chinese, especially women, cannot tolerate even small amounts physically. Some Chinese men drink hard liquor such as whisky and brandy.

BATHING

During certain periods such as illness, menses, and in the postpartum "sitting for the month" period, washing hair and bathing may be avoided. However, sponge baths are permissible. Infants may be bathed very frequently as cleanliness is highly valued.

AGEING

Chinese people value longevity. Old age is considered a time to enjoy the children and the harvest of fortune accumulated since youth. If elderly parents have children to care for them, this would be considered a life of good fortune.

Traditional responsibility for care of the elderly lies with the family and the oldest son and his wife; otherwise the unmarried children have the greatest obligation. Attending to and caring for the aged is a source of pride. It is extremely shameful for children to neglect their parents.

In Canada, elderly Chinese may be lonely or isolated because they lack English or other resources. Some parents expect them to perform household chores and care for the children while they go to work. Moreover, the younger generation who work may have little time to attend to the elderly. Elderly parents may expect care from their children, but those children may have adopted Western attitudes that the elderly should live independently and care for themselves.

Conflicts between the generations may arise over the best options for the elderly person who is ill. Old people may feel abandoned when placed in nursing homes, whereas their children may feel that this course is the best one for their parents.

DEATH AND DYING

Death is viewed as natural and inevitable. Families often prefer that health professionals not reveal the prognosis to dying patients, emphasizing that the patient's last days should be free of worry and pain. Postmortems may be refused by family members as they are viewed as unnecessarily invasive.

Mourning and funeral rites depend on the family's religion. There are, however, certain common Chinese rituals. Family members, relatives, and friends gather to mourn the deceased. Pregnant women, even if they are close family, are often not allowed to attend funerals for fear that sadness may harm their health. Female family members wear woollen flowers in their hair and males wear black armbands. Relatives of the deceased may not visit others for a certain period lest they bring bad luck.

DELIVERING CULTURALLY SENSITIVE HEALTH CARE

To offer culturally acceptable health care, professionals should be aware of several important characteristics among Chinese immigrants. Chinese people place great emphasis on work and education, values that influence their health and their use of health services. Professionals should be aware, too, of the traditional Chinese concepts of health and illness, especially the balance of yin and yang. This, in turn, helps explain the importance of food in maintaining health and treating illness.

Health professionals should be sensitive to their patients. Many Chinese seldom ask questions and thus need help in meeting Western expectations of the patient. Professionals should also be cognizant of the somatic ways in which clients portray illness, or the way they blame illness on external causes. They need furthermore to be informed of clients' perceptions of medications, treatment, and the general health care system.

Professionals should also be sensitive to the difficulties posed by the language barrier. Translators and other necessary resource persons should be carefully selected and utilized, and health care workers with experiences of Chinese people should be sought as consultants.

Although the family is an important resource, the self-sufficiency of the Chinese family should not be taken for granted. Nor should it be presumed that Chinese families do not need help in managing their problems. Family members should help to define areas of need and professionals should know of alternative forms of Chinese health care.

We have tried to present a picture of what Chinese people are like, but it should be clear that this community is very diverse. These people come from various geographic locations and socio-economic classes, and vary in culture, religion, beliefs, and experience. When we work with the Chinese, we must be aware of this diversity and avoid stereotyping at all costs. Instead, we should respect and acknowledge each person as a unique individual with a distinct background and values.

FURTHER READING

Chan, A. *Gold Mountain*. Vancouver, BC: New Star 1983

Employment and Immigration Canada. *Business Immigrants*. Ottawa: Minister of Supply and Services 1985

Gould-Marin, K. and N. Chorswnad. "Chinese Americans," in *Ethnicity and Medical Care*, ed. A. Harwood. Cambridge, MA: Harvard University Press 1981

Kleinman, A. *Patients and Healers in the Context of Culture*. Berkeley: University of California Press 1980

Kleinman, A. and Lin, T. *Normal and Abnormal Behavior in Chinese Culture*. Boston: Reidel 1981

Koo, L. "The use of food to treat and prevent disease in Chinese culture," *Social Science and Medicine*, Vol. 18, No. 9 (1984): 757–66

Lee, R.N.F. "The Chinese Perception of Mental Illness in the Canadian Mosaic," *Canada's Mental Health*, Vol. 34, No. 4 (1986): 2–4

Li, K.C. "The Chinese Perspective Towards Mental Illness and Its Implications in Treatment." Paper presented at Shaughnessy Hospital, Vancouver, BC (Feb. 1987)

Spector, R.E. *Cultural Diversity in Health and Illness*. New York: Appleton-Century Croft 1979

Starkins, E. "At First a Dream: One Hundred Years of Race Relations in Vancouver." Vancouver: Race Relations Adhoc Committee 1986

Statistics Canada. *Canada's Immigrants* (99–936). Ottawa: Minister of
   Supply and Services 1981a
— *Highlights: 1981 Census of Canada* (92-X-535E).
Ottawa: Census and Household Statistics Branch 1981b
Wong, G.F. Interview with Dr. G.F. Wong, former doctor of Chinese
   medicine in China. Vancouver, BC (Feb. 1987)

CONTRIBUTORS

Sharon Boyce (SUCCESS, Vancouver)
Raymond Chang (Strathcona Community Care Team, Vancouver)
Rita Kwan (SUCCESS, Vancouver)
David Lee (Ministry of Social Services and Housing, Vancouver)
Shirley Leung (SUCCESS, Vancouver)
K.C. Li (Strathcona Community Care Team, Vancouver)
Centina Low (SUCCESS, Vancouver)
Elaine Lui (Health Sciences Centre Hospital, UBC)
Margaret Ma (Vancouver, Health Department, North Unit)

CHAPTER FIVE

The Iranians

Afsaneh Behjati-Sabet

INTRODUCTION

Iranian immigrants comprise a steadily growing ethnic group in Canada, and many of them are settling in the Greater Vancouver area. The flow of people from Iran began in 1979, during and after the Islamic Revolution. Thus, most Iranians in Canada are first generation immigrants who share many of the beliefs, values, and characteristics of their compatriots in Iran.

Unlike the small number of Iranians who willingly migrated to North America, particularly the United States, before 1979, the majority of Iranians who have come to Canada since the Revolution left against their will and under tremendous pressure. Their flight has been from unbearable living conditions and religious and political persecution. Under these conditions it seems natural for the process of adjustment and integration to be slow. On the other hand, the vast majority of Iranians residing in Canada come from large urban areas and belong to upper and middle-class families, and are relatively familiar with Western education and values. Hence, the transition is probably smoother for this group of immigrants than for their counterparts from other countries. For this reason, the Iranian immigrant population of Canada is probably in a relatively advantageous position when dealing with Canadian public services, particularly medical and health services.

GEOGRAPHY AND HISTORY OF IRAN

Iran, formerly called Persia, is almost as large as the three western provinces of Canada combined and is mountainous in the north and west and low-lying in the centre and south. Bordering Iran to the north are Turkey, the USSR and the Caspian Sea. To the west are Turkey and Iraq, and to the East, Afghanistan and Pakistan. The Persian Gulf and the Sea of Oman separate southern Iran from the Arab Emirates and the Indian Ocean.

Iran's overall climate is affected by the two large deserts in the central and eastern regions, and is dry with high summer and low winter temperatures. The northern region bordering the Caspian and separated from the rest of the country by the Alborz mountains is, however, an exception and has a mild and humid climate with long rainy seasons. The southern coast is also very humid, but with much higher temperatures, far less rain, and longer summers.

Tehran, the capital, is situated in a dry area at the southern foot of the Alborz mountains and is known for its four distinct seasons. Most Iranian immigrants in Canada come from Tehran.

Iran has been classified as a developing country and is basically an agricultural society which produces rice, wheat, tea, cotton, citrus fruits, and dried fruits. It is one of the world's largest oil producers and a powerful member of OPEC.

The very rapid growth of the oil industry since the turn of the century, and its nationalization in the 1950s, dramatically increased per capita income in Iran and encouraged rapid technological growth. Large urban areas developed and migration to cities occurred on a large scale. This in turn deepened national class divisions.

Iran has a population of approximately forty million, mainly of Indo-European race. However, a large population of ethnic Turks, Kurds, and Arabs lives in the northern, western, and southern border areas. Also, many nomadic tribes are spread throughout Iran and they migrate from place to place twice a year, supporting themselves by sheep- and cattle-raising. Among these tribal families are the Bakhtiaris, Ghashghais, and the Turkomans. Each tribe has its own distinctive characteristics, customs, dialects, and styles of dress. Within the last few decades some tribal members and families have migrated to large urban areas or travelled abroad, mainly to receive higher education. These tribal members tend to retain most of their cultural heritage and, at the same time, live modern, semi-Western lifestyles. For example, they adopt Western dress, travel widely, and are ambitious and well-educated, but maintain strong ties with their nomadic kinsfolk, by whom they are highly revered. Any Iranian Canadians of tribal background are most likely to belong to this group.

The populations of Tehran and other large cities have increased since the outbreak of the Iran-Iraq War in 1980, which left millions homeless in the southwestern regions of Iran. This bloody war, which ended in 1988, was a major reason for the flight of many Iranians to Western countries.

While the Persian culture goes back many thousands of years a written account of the history of Persia only dates from 559 BC. During the course of its history, Iran (or Persia) has experienced several invasions and has consequently absorbed various cultures which have laid the basis of modern Iranian society.

The most important invasion was the Arab conquest in the seventh century which put an end to the last of three great pre-Islamic dynasties and extinguished the predominantly Zoroastrian society. The Islamization of Persia took place very rapidly and Islam has since been the major religion of the country. Currently 98 per cent of the Iranian population is Moslem, of which 93 per cent belong to the Shi'ite sect (Jalali 1982). In fact, it is Shi'ism which differentiates Iranians from most of the Moslem world, which is Sunni.

After the lengthy fight for independence from the Islamic Caliphate was won, Persia experienced several centuries of strict Islamic rule, under a number of dynasties. Consequently, religious rules became the governing laws of Iran. A system of constitutional monarchy was established around the turn of the twentieth century. However, the constitutional dimension of the system remained largely nominal, and Iran continued to fall under the undisputed power of the Shahs (kings). The last monarch was Muhammad Reza of the Pahlavi dynasty who reigned for thirty-seven years (1941–79) and was overthrown in the Islamic Revolution led by Ayatollah Khomeini. The Islamic Republic of Iran was established with a strict, fundamentalist Islamic regime in control.

During the reign of the Pahlavi family (1925–79) some attempts at modernization were made. Universities were established and students were sent abroad by the government to acquire higher education. The "Unveiling Act" was enacted in 1937 as the first step towards the emancipation of women. Women were given voting rights in the 1960s. Western lifestyles and values became more prevalent.

Since 1979 the trend in Iran has been towards a much more traditional and religious lifestyle. This has made living conditions generally unbearable for a majority of the rapidly emerging educated and Westernized upper and middle-classes, the modern women in particular. Moreover, the lengthy and bloody war between Iran and its neighbour, Iraq, exacted unbelievable human and economic casualties and evoked the constant fear of conscription in thousands of young boys and men. Added to this has been the never-ending persecution of various political, ideological, and religious groups and the well-documented violation of human rights. All these factors constitute the most important reasons for Iranian migration to Western countries, especially Canada and the United States, since 1979.

LANGUAGE

The spoken and written official language of Iran is Farsi or Persian, a language that is over 1,000 years old. The Farsi script is Arabic. Since the Arab conquest and the Islamization of Persia in the seventh century, Farsi has been profoundly influenced by Arabic although it has remained distinctly different from Arabic. The Arab population on the Iran-Iraq border and near the Persian Gulf speak Arabic and the Turks along the border with Turkey speak a dialect of Turkish. Each tribal group speaks its own dialect.

SOCIAL CLASS STRUCTURE

The majority of Iranians residing in Canada belong to the more modern, educated, and affluent urban classes and tend to differ from their compatriots in many respects. At the same time they share common characteristics that could be considered very "Persian." Iranians are a very class-conscious people and class is a central factor in Iranian society. Health professionals will find it much easier and more effective to work with Iranian patients if they are sensitive to the importance of the distinct, identifiable elements. Some of these elements of Iran's social class structure are discussed below.

TRADITIONAL SOCIETY

While the majority of the Iranian population is rural (60–5 per cent) and illiterate (approximately 65 per cent), the urban population is much more varied and can be divided into several classes: lower, traditional middle, modernized middle, and upper. The latter two groups are most heavily represented in Canada.

The traditional middle class consists of affluent, very religious Moslem families. Today's religious leaders (the clergy) and political leaders belong to this class. For many decades this class has controlled Iran's economy, as well as its political, religious, and ideological life. Sometimes this control has had to be subtle and stealthy.

RELIGIOUS SUBGROUPS

The 2 per cent of the population which is not Moslem probably belongs to the more modern middle class. In this group are the Baha'i, the largest minority with about half a million members, Zoroastrians, Jews, and Christians, comprising Armenians and Assyrians. The Baha'i faith is the only one among the subgroups mentioned above that is not officially recognized in Iran. Some intolerance towards the other subgroups exists, and Iran has always been rated quite low in religious tolerance. It should be noted that politics and religion are two very sensitive aspects in an Iranian's life and much tact is required when dealing with them.

Due to the strong class-consciousness prevailing in the Iranian society, members of upper and lower classes do not usually interact socially. For example, intermarriage is uncommon. The same attitude prevails between religious and political groupings. However, due to the expansion of free education at all levels and its accessibility to larger numbers of Iranians from all social strata, class mobility has become both possible and very common. Iranians in Canada tend to confine themselves to their own social class (which is defined mainly by levels of affluence and education), their own religious groups, and to those who share the same political views.

In order to help patients adjust to life in Canada, some health professionals may encourage friendships between their Iranian patients or may refer them to an Iranian professional. The helpful professional must be sensitive to the diversity mentioned above. For example, a Canadian physician recounts how she once tried to establish contact between two of her female Iranian patients in order to help one of them overcome her severe isolation and loneliness. The patient immediately reacted with the question, "Which political group does this other person belong to?", a question which the physician could not answer. Or, a female Baha'i counsellor recalls trying to establish rapport with a depressive male Moslem client who had been referred to her by a Canadian professional solely on the basis of shared homeland and language. The client did not return after the first interview and the counsellor's attempts to establish further contact failed completely.

BASIC NATIONAL AND CULTURAL CHARACTERISTICS

Regardless of the regional, ethnic, religious, and social class diversity among Iranians, all have some cultural characteristics in common.

These were perhaps developed to ensure Persian self-preservation in the face of political turmoil and instability over many centuries. Even though Iranians have absorbed cultural traits from successive waves of invaders, they have managed to maintain their own sense of uniqueness and identity.

This is the source of much pride, and Iranians are nostalgically tied to the past. For an Iranian, loss of Persian identity is shameful. This strong sense of uniqueness and pride makes for a people who dislike admitting their smallest mistakes for fear of losing face (Zonis 1976; Graham 1978). For example, it is very common for Iranians to deny material losses or financial needs, and to pretend the opposite. North Americans are often deceived by the well-groomed appearance of Iranians and it is sometimes difficult for them to believe that the person may indeed be suffering financially.

Iranians have also been characterized as suspicious, distrustful, and somewhat cynical (Zonis 1976; Graham 1978). This sense of distrust is apparent in their dealings outside the circle of family and close friends. Cynicism and distrust also typify the Iranian's dealings with government authorities and the Western world, both of which are believed to have exploited the Persian nation (Graham 1978). Underlying all this is a sense of insecurity associated with years of political unrest and upheaval.

Trust and submission are openly expressed and exercised only towards God and one's family and friends (Nyrop 1978). Family members and close friends will literally sacrifice for one another. Family ties are strong and it is one's duty to keep, at all times, the good name of the family (Nyrop 1978; Haeri 1980).

Submission to God's will is an even more important aspect of an Iranian's life. Although this attitude has recently waned among the educated who are more likely to assume individual responsibility for their own lives, the deep-rooted cultural belief in fate or "Taghdir" remains strong in all classes. Iranians are expected to accept life's events and consequences with grace, based on the belief that "all is in the mighty hands of God." Because of their pride and competitiveness, Iranians residing in Canada suffer greatly from a sense of lost status and social rank. Canadians may notice that Iranian immigrants enjoy boasting—with much enthusiasm—about their glamorous past. Perhaps this is an attempt to be accepted and understood by the mainstream society. Possibly, in attempting to conceal the losses, which they are expected to accept gracefully, and satisfy their pride, many Iranians in the West develop various psychosomatic disorders.

The Western preoccupation with punctuality is not shared by Iranians who almost always take their time to socialize and establish personal relationships before getting down to business. For example, an Iranian patient prefers to spend the first five or ten minutes of an appointment exchanging informal and personal information with the doctor. Iranians conduct their business affairs along similar lines and many contracts are initiated and informally closed during social gatherings. This social ritual may sometimes annoy health and social service professionals who are pressed for time. Keeping appointments and punctuality are other potential areas of conflict with Iranian patients. Some health professionals in Canada recount how Iranian patients have arrived late for appointments or have cancelled them at the last minute.

Touching, embracing, and kissing are very common among persons of the same sex and conversational distance for Iranians is usually less than for North Americans. Eye contact may be far less than is typical for North Americans.

FAMILY STRUCTURE

The family is the most important element in Iranian culture and life is usually dominated by family values and relationships. Reliance on family connections for influence, employment, and security still holds true and is very common in all classes. Iranians in Canada who are generally unfamiliar with the Western individualism find it difficult to adjust to the loss of connections.

The extended family has traditionally been the basic unit of society and has retained its social and psychological bonds despite the recent relative growth of nuclear families in urban areas. In fact, the word "family" in Persian refers to the extended family and an Iranian is usually judged by the name of his or her family, including grandparents, aunts, uncles, and cousins.

While sharing some universal and basic characteristics, Iranian families can be classified into two major groups—traditional and modern (Jalali 1982).

Traditional Family Structure

Among Iranians currently living in Canada, very few belong to traditional families. However, this family structure is discussed here to provide a broader perspective on Iranian society and to describe the original lifestyle of those few traditional families which do exist in

Canada. Most of the original practices and living arrangements disappear when these families move to the West but many of the values
may persist.

The traditional Iranian family is a strong patriarchal unit whose
undisputed head is the oldest male of the extended family, all of
whose members live together in the same household. The family
consists of husband and wife—some men have up to four wives—
unmarried children, married sons, and their wives and children. The
father has authority over the entire family and is responsible for the
discipline of all his children and grandchildren. The wife's role is to
submit to her husband. However, she is very close to her children
and should conflicts arise between father and children, she usually
intervenes.

Marriages are usually arranged. The couple's fathers negotiate the
exchange of dowry, property, and jewellery, and the prospective
couple have very little basic say in the matter. A bond of marriage is
considered a strong, unifying tie between the two families, and is
never to be broken (Jalali 1982). Divorce is very rare, but does exist
and the woman usually returns to her own family leaving her children behind. The daughter-in-law must submit to her husband's
mother and any older sisters. Chastity is highly revered and premarital sexual activities are considered sinful, especially for women. Un-
chaste single women in traditional families are harshly stigmatized.

Modern Family Structure

Modern families from middle- and upper-class urban Iran are most
often represented in the Iranian immigrant population of Canada.
These families hold many Western values and follow some Western
life patterns. For example, among the major effects of Westernization
on Iranian families have been the weakening of parental authority,
the much increased freedom of marital choice and the consequent
development of the nuclear family. Single men continue to live with
their parents, but married men are expected to live in separate
households with their wives and children. Father continues to be the
major bread-winner and the head of the household, though he has diminished power and authority. While the Muslim religion allows men
to take several wives, this practice has fallen into virtual abeyance.

Western education and foreign travel have changed the woman's
role drastically. In Iran, since the 1960s, many women have entered
the work-force and more women are seeking higher education; by
1979 about 40 per cent of all university students in Iran were
women. Women typically marry between twenty-two and twenty-

five, unlike traditional families where most women are married between fifteen and eighteen (Jalali 1982). More and more single women from modern families postpone marriage, which generally is no longer arranged, for the sake of better education. Iranian women are generally five to ten years younger than their husbands.

Premarital sexual activities, although not uncommon, are considered sinful in modern families, whose attitude towards chastity is only slightly more open than that of traditional families. Sex before marriage is more acceptable for men and is much less common among young women. The level of tolerance of, and openness to, premarital sex seems to have increased slightly among Iranians residing in Canada.

The breakdown of the extended family, greater employment opportunities for women, increased marriage age, higher living standards, and the preoccupation with better education have all led to a decrease in the number of children in nuclear families to two or three. Even though women have become emancipated and educated and have acquired more decision-making power in the home and out, the modern Iranian family remains a patriarchal unit in which sex roles are almost immune to change. This means that modern Iranian women are expected to take on most household responsibilities and maintain outside jobs.

Two major characteristics shared by families of all classes are the value placed on extended family advice and support, for example, regarding major health problems, and the respect and dutifulness shown the elderly. For example, the health professional may frequently be called by not just one but several of the patient's relatives to explain the results of a medical test. Or should the physician recommend an operation, the same number of persons expect to be consulted by the patient and his or her family before consent is given. The deep sense of duty towards the elderly includes responsibility for the care of old and dying family members. There are very few nursing homes in Iran and sending elderly people to them is considered disrespectful and cruel. If families do place their elderly in Canadian nursing homes they tend to interfere with the nursing home's management of the old person.

MIGRATION TO CANADA

Although some Iranian families settled in eastern Canada in the 1960s and 1970s, there has only been one major migration wave from Iran to Canada since 1979. Toronto and Vancouver have absorbed the majority of Iranian immigrants. According to immigration officials, close to 8,000 Iranians currently reside in BC, mostly in the Greater Vancouver area, particularly the North Shore.

The most important reasons for migration have been, and continue to be, the political, religious, and economic situation in Iran, together with the consequences and dangers of the recent war in the Persian Gulf. Most Iranians come from the urban upper and middle-classes but they differ among themselves in politics, religion and ideology. Opposition political leaders and members (including those of the Islamic group, Mujjahedin), high ranking officials of the Shah's regime, less traditional Moslems, and members of all the religious minorities make up the majority of immigrants or refugees. Even though social interaction between groups does occur, there is a strong tendency for members of each subgroup to stick together.

SOCIO-ECONOMIC STATUS IN CANADA

Most men hold university degrees, some at doctoral level, and come from various professional and business backgrounds. Of those who have come with investment capital, many have established small businesses, particularly in real estate.

Women, on the other hand, generally have a lower level of education, having usually only finished high school or bachelor's degrees. The younger generation of Iranian women in Canada (late twenties to early forties) have generally obtained post-secondary degrees and have been employed in Iran, mainly in the traditional areas of nursing, teaching, administration, and the arts. There are a number of female medical doctors residing in British Columbia, very few of whom practice medicine.

Most Iranian immigrants must live and work under conditions lower than they expected or were used to. Since most, if not all, belong to upper and middle income families with professional backgrounds and higher status, unemployment and taking manual jobs represent challenges which are difficult to meet. Since 1984, over 90 per cent of Iranians who arrived in Canada as refugees (government-sponsored or otherwise), have received social assistance. This can be very degrading for the proud Iranian and may account for many of the physical and emotional problems that health professionals frequently encounter.

SPECIAL PROBLEMS IN CANADA

The major problems faced by Iranians in Canada are unemployment, underemployment, loss of status, and financial loss, in short, downward socio-economic mobility. Other factors compound this problem, including language barriers and an underlying suspicion of Western culture.

Fluency in any foreign language, of course, goes beyond the mere knowledge of that language and embraces a vast area of cultural values and meanings. Iranian immigrants, the men in particular, have entered Canada with some knowledge of English (or French in the older generation). However, most Iranians do not communicate easily in English with non-Persian speaking persons. They simply do not understand the intent behind verbal messages. These factors place an Iranian at a disadvantage when, for example, applying for a job.

For women and the elderly the problem of language is even greater, since they tend to be more isolated and to have fewer opportunities to master English.

Another major factor contributing to loss of status and un- or underemployment in Canada's Iranian community is its attitude towards the North American culture. Iranians, in general, are fearful of Western influences, especially on their children. They do not approve of the permissiveness that they see in mainstream Canadian society. Moreover, they are nostalgic about their past and their cultural identity, fear change, and distrust outsiders. Consequently, to protect themselves and their youngsters they isolate themselves and maintain few social contacts with Canadian society at large. Some religious subgroups may differ; Baha'is and Christians, for example, are generally more sociable and even intermarry with the mainstream population. The levels of familiarity with mainstream patterns of life and work are very low, sometimes to the extent of keeping Iranians in ignorance of their rights and the services available to them. For example, they may know little or nothing about the Human Rights Commission, free legal aid services, unemployment insurance, and other social services. However, Iranians trust and use most branches of the health services in Canada, with the exception of the mental health services.

In the Iranian families in Canada, generation gaps and conflicts tend to increase. Children, usually the first ones to learn English and lose their mother tongue, grow farther and farther apart from their families. Communication breakdown is common. The tendency to shelter and protect children from Western influences and values is strong. At the same time, Iranian children, both male and female, are expected to do extraordinarily well at school. Iranian parents expect their children to achieve high marks but to avoid integration into the larger society. These conflicting standards lead to a great deal of family discord, and sometimes to rebellion on the part of the children.

Expectations about sexual roles are another potential area of family conflict. For decades in Iran, modern women have had to struggle, usually successfully, to hold jobs both in and out of the home. In Canada, however, many are forced to fulfil a new role. They have now become bread-winners, in some cases sole bread-winners, on whose shoulders rests the financial well-being of the family. As a result, the man's lowered self-esteem, because of loss of status, position, and possessions, falls even further. Men tend to lose face and conflicts arise. In addition, due to the loss of the extended family's help and the lack of domestic servants, men find themselves having to share the unfamiliar duties of child-rearing and housekeeping with their wives.

All the above factors, together with a general increase in the women's awareness of their rights to independence, have led to a drastic increase in the rate of separation and divorce in Iranian immigrant families. In Iran, divorce carries a great deal of stigma, for both men and women; however, the female partner generally suffers more. According to Islam, men take custody of the children, who are then raised by the father's family. For women, lack of financial independence and loss of face in the community make divorce much harder to accept. However, Iranian women from broken marriages are supported by their original families and return to them in cases of separation or divorce. This tradition is well maintained in Canada for those who, of course, have an extended family accessible to them. Women with no extended families in Canada usually live on their own after having achieved some financial security through employment, court rulings, or social assistance.

ADDITIONAL NOTES ON IRANIANS IN CANADA

Most Iranian families residing in Canada are nuclear families. Nevertheless, when grandparents do join families in Canada, they usually live with their children for reasons of financial and emotional support. This is particularly true in the case of very old grandparents. Although the elderly are the most respected members of the family, their son or son-in-law remains the head of the family and shares his decision-making rights with his wife.

Major decisions such as property or business purchases or the children's education are usually made jointly by husband and wife. The actual implementation of plans and decisions, however, is the husband's prerogative as he has overall control of family possessions. This, of course, does not completely deprive the woman of authority over money, whether hers or the family's, and most Iranian women seem to enjoy a fair amount of freedom in spending money. Most of the shopping, for example, is done and controlled by women.

In an Iranian family, the children are the least respected and enjoy limited freedom. Unmarried children of any age and of both sexes usually live with the family and move out only after they are married. Marriages are not arranged and children have the last word in choice of partner. Nevertheless, parental consent is essential to the decision. Dating is allowed but with limitations. Boys are usually given more freedom to date than girls and dating generally begins at a later age than for Canadian youth. Iranian parents definitely prefer their sons and daughters to date and mingle with those they know well and trust, preferably other Iranians. Children gain more freedom as they grow older. However, sex before marriage remains unacceptable at any age, particularly for girls. Family reputation, affluence, education, and physical appearance are the most important considerations in choosing marriage partners. Children, particularly young women, are expected at all times to safeguard the good name of the family. This attitude has led to communication breakdowns and generational divisions within Iranian families living in Canada.

Since children have very little say in major family decisions, they are usually not consulted and communication between parents and their offspring remains minimal. Discussion of sex in the family is a definite taboo. Children are also usually kept in the dark about the family's financial and emotional problems. This is generally done in an attempt to protect the children.

Family violence is generally low. The rate of physical and sexual abuse of children is in the lower range. Discipline (e.g., spanking) is usually administered by the father (and may be harsher than the Canadian norm), since the mother is considered the more loving, caring, and protective figure in the family. Verbal abuse of children, on the other hand, may be common. Wife battering is not known to be common, perhaps as a result of the extreme importance Iranians place on family reticence.

Problem-solving and conflict resolution usually occur in stages and according to a certain pattern. Every effort is made to keep a problem private. Should the parties involved (e.g., marriage partners, in-laws, business partners) fail to resolve the conflict, often the case because of the extreme emotionalism of those involved, a third party is asked to intervene impartially. This person will be trusted and respected by both sides, usually an elderly man well known and respected in the community. Reconciliation happens on the basis of "forgive and forget" and the problem is never mentioned again, whether it is truly resolved or not. Professional help, be it from a counsellor, physician, lawyer, or the courts is only reluctantly sought as a last resort. This attitude may account for the delays, at times extreme, in reporting incidents of family violence, attempted suicide, or mental and emotional problems to professionals. It should be noted, however, that if Iranians do seek professional help, they generally prefer to be referred to non-Iranian professionals to preserve confidentiality and face.

Iranians are generally not very familiar with the leisure services provided in Canada. In Iran, community sports were not very common and costly activities such as skiing, swimming, tennis, and so on, were available only to the elite. Iranian children in Canadian schools may be less active in sports and other extracurricular activities since the family usually emphasizes academic achievement. The school system may have little difficulty in involving Iranian parents in their children's academic work, but greater difficulty in eliciting parental participation in extracurricular activities. This trend, however, is changing and more Iranians are realizing the importance of physical and social activities for their children. By the same token, more and more Iranian families are becoming physically and socially active.

Leisure time, for the most part, is spent as family time. Visiting relatives and friends, mostly Iranian, for many hours at a time, and eating extravagant Persian dishes is the commonest way of socializing, and children are almost always present. An Iranian party usually consists of three or four generations gathered together. Using baby-sitters (and daycare, for that matter) is rather uncommon and children are usually kept up until late at night.

Hospitality is one of the most important features of the Persian culture and a source of much pride. Persian hospitality is characterized by extreme generosity in the sharing of food. The offering and receiving of food (or gifts) is done according to a certain ritual called "taarof," which symbolizes courtesy and good manners. Once an Iranian is offered something he or she is expected to reject it gracefully for a few times before finally accepting it from the other party, who is in turn expected to persist in his or her generous offers. Refusing food from an Iranian causes offence and may be perceived as rejection.

Health professionals who may have been offered dinner invitations or gifts of specially prepared Persian dishes should regard them as tokens of appreciation and respect and, whenever possible, should accept them after some "taarof." However, they should be aware that once they have gained the trust of their Iranian patients they may be called upon for minor favours; this was the normal pattern in Iran. For example, paediatricians in Canada recount incidents where adult family members have asked for help and advice about their own minor health concerns or personal problems while the paediatrician is busy treating the child.

HEALTH AND HEALTH PRACTICES

In the past forty or fifty years the Iranian people, particularly the urban populations, have rapidly become familiar with Western medicine and health care, and have generally trusted and respected it. Nevertheless, some folk beliefs and traditions are retained and occasionally practised.

Iranian immigrants generally do not refute scientific theories about underlying causes of diseases. However, coming from a fatalistic society, as they do, may place them side by side with their strong belief in the will of God, especially in the event of death. The belief that "all is in the mighty hands of God," however, does not prevent an Iranian from seeing a physician for help when needed.

Food and other natural substances are believed to play a role in health and Iranians are known to seek constant guidance from physicians about their children's diets. To keep their children healthy and robust—for thin children are not considered healthy—Iranians tend to overfeed them and to become overly concerned about poor appetites. The use of "hot" and "cold" foods to prevent or cure minor illnesses is also common. Certain foods such as honey, sugar, and nuts are considered hot, whereas yogurt, berries, and watermelon are considered cold. Consuming too much of one and too little of the other is believed to cause stomach upsets or other minor disorders. When minor ailments such as low fever or cold symptoms occur, an effort is made to cure them at home with the help of food and herbs. Should the illness persist, the doctor is called. Delays in seeking medical help, with the exception of psychiatrists, are not a major problem among Iranians.

In pre-revolutionary Iran there were about 12,000 physicians; about one-quarter of these practised in Tehran and the remainder in other large cities. Rural health services were poor and most rural people relied on traditional and non-professional healers. Medical insurance is not universal in Iran and government health services lacked and still lack quality. Therefore medical help is sought from physicians in private practice only when illness persists and only by those who can afford the cost. Families choose one general practitioner whom they and their relatives know and trust and with whom they establish close relationships. Family doctors become the confidants of their patients and have detailed knowledge of their patients' personal lives. Appointments to see a physician are often made directly by the patient or the patient's mother in the case of young children. An elderly person is usually accompanied by his or her child.

The fact that Iranians had direct access to specialists in Iran has become a problem in Canada where a GP must refer patients to specialists. Iranians in Canada sometimes seek alternative routes for making appointments with specialists. For example, an Iranian paediatrician in Vancouver constantly receives telephone calls from Iranian acquaintances asking him to arrange appointments with other specialists. This is done because Iranian patients fear giving offence to their family doctor by requesting referrals to specialists.

PREVALENCE OF DISEASE IN IRAN

Due to the expansion in Iran of free vaccination services, running water, and inter-regional communication in the last few decades, the rate of infant mortality has dropped drastically in most areas of the country. Life expectancy has risen from age forty in the 1940s, to fifty-eight in 1981. Thus, the population of Iran has tripled in the last forty years.

Diseases specific to warm climatic regions used to be prevalent in the country, but almost all of these have been successfully controlled. However, cases of typhoid and para-typhoid were reported in some areas of Iran after the outbreak of the Iran-Iraq war. Also, gradual loss of hearing due to early childhood illnesses may require attention from Canadian health professionals working with Iranians over the age of fifty.

PREVALENCE OF DISEASE IN CANADA

Health consciousness is a rather important feature of the Iranian population in Canada. This may be accounted for by the fact that Iranians as a group do not present the health professionals with typical diseases. However, physicians working with Iranian immigrants and students have recounted many cases of psychosomatic disorders and stress-related depressions, which are known to be more common among women and middle-aged men. Loss of career and status is probably a major reason for the phenomenon. Because Iranians residing in Canada are proud people and come from predominantly professional, educated, and affluent backgrounds, they find it difficult to cope with the losses they experience in Canada. These stresses lead to physical and mental symptoms.

MENTAL ILLNESS

Iranians generally resist seeking help from psychiatrists and other professionals in mental health agencies, mainly because of the stigma associated with mental illness. In the educated middle and upper classes mental illness is often attributed to heredity or physical dysfunction (e.g., dysfunctions of the nervous system). Many people in Iran also attribute insanity to evil spirits. The majority of families tend to conceal such problems for fear of jeopardizing their children's chances of marriage (Lipson and Meleis 1983). Often, a person may be very sick indeed before the psychiatrist's help is finally sought.

Iranians are much more comfortable with physical than with mental illnesses. The first reaction of many Iranians to a diagnosis requiring mental health treatment is denial. For this reason the help of neurologists is often sought when emotional health problems arise. For the same reason, medication is more readily accepted that non-biomedical treatment. A very small minority of the Iranians with emotional problems may prefer counsellors and psychotherapists to medical doctors.

RELATIONSHIP BETWEEN PATIENT AND PROFESSIONAL

In general, Iranian patients seek a more personal relationship with their doctors than do mainstream Canadians. They expect their physicians to listen to long stories about their health and personal problems. Also, they expect a great deal of understanding since they regard family doctors as confidants. Iranians also like to be given time to boast about their past accomplishments, careers, and lifestyles or their high status and rank in Iranian society. In order for a Canadian physician to gain his or her Iranian patient's confidence and trust, he or she must take the time to listen and respond sympathetically, undertake full and thorough examinations, and devote undivided attention to the patient during an appointment. Trust can be established during the first few visits and once this is achieved, the patient becomes a "believer" in his or her doctor. This is a notion commonly held by Iranians, and once fulfilled, will very likely cause the patient to follow the physician's advice. Trusted and "believed in" doctors are regarded as definite authorities, or parental figures, and older male doctors are more readily trusted. Initial choice of family doctor is usually made on the basis of personal recommendations from more experienced friends and relatives. Upon first arriving in Canada Iranians may rush from one doctor to another in an attempt to find the one most suited to them.

Although Iranians are a talkative group of people, some probing seems to be useful in helping Iranian patients overcome initial shyness and distrust. Iranians who have not followed the physician's advice such as abstaining from certain foods, might at times try to conceal the truth, usually in an attempt not to lose the respect of their doctor.

X-rays and blood tests are popular with Iranian patients, who are rather impatient about hearing the test results from their doctors. They prefer immediate answers and often telephone the physician for quick results. Iranians may also become very impatient when asked to wait for any length of time before seeing specialists.

Since preventative care is generally not practised in Iran, many patients may complain that "the doctors didn't do anything" when medication is not prescribed. Pills and injections are most popular; injections are believed to render faster results. A physician residing in Canada who had practised for over thirty years in Tehran recounts several incidents in which his patients refused to pay for the hour-long visits on the grounds that he had "only talked" and had not prescribed any kind of medicine. Expensive and rare drugs are preferred to ordinary pills, and doctors who prescribe the most expensive ones are regarded as the most skilled. Many young families, however, have changed their attitudes about medicine and the above tradition is changing steadily.

Since Iranians belong to a strongly patriarchal society, it is only natural that male physicians are trusted and esteemed more than their female counterparts. Moreover, the older the physician, the greater the trust and respect. Female doctors, however, are trusted equally, even preferred, in certain areas of medicine. Women gynaecologists and obstetricians, pediatricians and eye specialists are preferred, whereas female neurosurgeons, for example, may be regarded by Iranians as unworthy of trust. (Almost one-third of medical students in Iran are women, most of whom graduate in gynaecology, paediatrics, and obstetrics.) Generally Iranian men prefer seeing a male physician to a female one (Jalali 1982).

HOSPITALIZATION

Iranians are very sociable and hospital visits to friends or relatives are considered a moral duty. Visitors come in large numbers, bring sweets, flowers, and gifts, and stay for long hours. For them it is a time to socialize and to keep the patient company. Iranians have a tendency to disregard hospital regulations about visiting hours, staying with the patient overnight or bringing forbidden food. Close family members, for example a mother or a spouse, are known to make extraordinary demands on hospital workers and to interfere with their handling of the patient. For example, an Iranian mother whose child is hospitalized may ask to stay with her child at all times, protest at the quality of food, and request and expect special treatment for her child. Or she may want to bathe the child and change his or her linen herself.

Should these problems arise, asking the family doctor or a trusted specialist to intervene gently may be the most effective solution. It should be noted, though, that most hospitalized Iranians enjoy having large numbers of noisy visitors and should be allowed to receive them if health and hospital regulations permit. Wherever possible, Iranian patients prefer to stay in private hospital rooms.

Nurses are regarded highly by Iranians. However, they are given little respect when in the presence of a physician. Messages that come from a doctor are much more readily obeyed. Iranian women may experience great discomfort in the presence of male nurses. Whenever possible, female nurses should be used.

MEDICATION AND TREATMENT

Drugs are the preferred means of treatment among Iranians and physicians in Canada will have little difficulty in convincing Iranian patients to take prescribed medication. However, convincing an Iranian to exercise regularly or to cut down on certain foods may be a different matter. Iranians often promise to follow their doctors' advice on physical activity and dietary habits, but seldom succeed in doing so.

REHABILITATION

Like mental illness, mental and physical handicaps are stigmatized in Iran. Most kinds of prenatal and perinatal disabilities are viewed as hereditary and hence are concealed from the eyes of the public. Although this trend is changing among the educated middle classes, all Iranians become uncomfortable in the presence of disabled and mentally handicapped persons. Many fear that the handicap may run in the family and pity the victim and the family. This attitude, combined with the shame and pity felt by the victim's own family almost always results in depression in the victim, isolation, and sometimes suicide.

In Iran, the deaf and blind are the least stigmatized, and the mentally retarded the most. Those disabled later in life suffer less stigma but probably the same amount of pity. Because of Iranian attitudes to disability, and the scarcity of rehabilitation and self-care services in Iran (with the exception of those for the blind), mentally and physically disabled individuals in Iran lack the motivation to adapt. Rehabilitation professionals in Canada may find working with Iranian clients and their families extremely difficult.

FAMILY PLANNING

Families in rural Iran are much larger (up to twelve children) than those in urban areas and the average size of modern middle-class families in Iran has shrunk to four or five within the last few decades. In Canada, most young Iranian families do not have more than two or three children. Birth control, although forbidden by Islam, is practised by almost all Iranian families in Canada. The favourite methods of contraception, generally chosen by women, are birth control pills and the IUD.

Couples generally plan to have their first child within the first three years of marriage. Since children are regarded as blessings and procreation is considered the major reason for marriage, family pressures on couples increase when the first pregnancy is delayed. The second child usually follows within two to three years and it is not uncommon for couples to wait for many years before having a third child. Male children are generally preferred. This preference is especially strong among Jews and quite strong among Moslems.

Abortions are illegal in Iran and take place only for medical reasons in an attempt to save the life of the mother. However, illegality had not lowered the abortion rate in urban areas before the Revolution. Many legal, illegal, professional, and non-professional abortions took place in hospitals, clinics, and homes. Frequency of abortions among Iranian women may not be as high as that for Canadian women, but Iranian women from all denominations do occasionally seek help to terminate unwanted pregnancies.

Since premarital sex is considered taboo, a pregnant single woman may be harshly ostracized, particularly in rural Iran. Educated middle-class families often seek abortions in complete secrecy. Illegitimate infants are usually put up for adoption or into an orphanage. Pregnancies out of wedlock cause intense crisis and turmoil in Iranian families, regardless of class.

PREGNANCY AND PRENATAL CARE

Pregnancy is considered a blessing and expectant Iranian women become the focus of much attention and care. The traditional belief among all classes of Iranians is that pregnant women must abstain from heavy physical work, rest frequently, and eat rich and healthy foods. Extensive weight gain often becomes a problem. Exposure to Western medicine has changed this trend to a certain degree. Nevertheless health professionals in Canada may encounter difficulty in convincing pregnant Iranian women to exercise regularly. In Canada, the majority of Iranian women and their husbands attend prenatal classes. However, not all the advice given in class is followed.

Because of the relatively high level of education among younger Iranian women in Canada, they generally recognize early signs of pregnancy and therefore go to the doctor at an early stage. Husbands and mothers of the pregnant woman are the first family members to be informed. Information about pregnancy is passed on from mother to daughter or daughter-in-law, usually immediately after the onset of pregnancy.

CHILDBIRTH AND POSTPARTUM PERIOD

In Iran, childbirth takes place in hospitals, private clinics, and in homes, and the delivery is attended by physicians and certified midwives. Close female relatives keep mothers company at childbirth. In Canada, more and more Iranian fathers are now present in delivery rooms.

Iranian women express their pain and anguish in labour more freely and loudly than their Canadian counterparts. Screaming and sobbing are considered normal when giving birth. In fact, women are encouraged to scream loudly and freely. Some Iranian women may find the pain unbearable and it is common for them to ask for an anaesthetic.

In Iran infants are brought to their mothers only to be breast-fed, since new mothers are believed to need rest and quiet. Extended family members are always available to provide help in the early weeks after birth and the new mother is either taken to her parents' home or joined by her mother. Certain foods such as barley, and water drained from boiling rice are considered good for increasing the milk flow and mothers are fed these and other rich foods. In Canada, breast-feeding usually lasts for nine months to a year. The length of this period, however, may change according to the mother's work and health. Iranian mothers have no difficulty in using substitute formulas.

Visiting the new mother and her baby is common practice among Iranians. The mother and infant are not secluded and usually begin socializing outside the home within two or three weeks of childbirth. Regular visits by public health nurses in Canada are highly valued by Iranian women who, although unfamiliar with the idea, fully appreciate the information and support they receive. Most new mothers need and use this education on child care in Canada and on the resources available to them.

DEATH AND DYING

"God gives life and God takes life." This belief is commonly held by almost all Iranians. For this reason members of a dying person's family do not plan for death. By the same token, they never give up hope, not even after doctors have pronounced that the patient is dying. Grief is not permitted in the presence of the dying patient for fear of weakening the person's will to live. Death, as near as it may be, is never openly discussed. Plans for the funeral and mourning are made only after death has occurred. It is believed to be best to die at home in the presence of the whole family, for dying in loneliness and solitude is disgraceful.

Moslems in Iran do not use coffins to bury their dead. Because of this, some Moslem Iranians have difficulty with burial practices in Canada. Most Iranian religious sects prescribe certain bathing rituals for the dead, and a majority of Iranians here ask to bathe their dead accordingly. Funerals may be held on the same day as the death or several days after. It is often preferred that the body be kept in the hospital before burial. Cremation is most uncommon among all Iranian subgroups, who bury their dead according to their own religious ceremonies.

Once death occurs, mourning is loud. In fact, men and especially women are expected to sob loudly and even to overreact. Visits of condolence are a moral obligation for all relatives, friends, and even acquaintances. Memorial services are held at the time of the funeral as well as several days later; for example, Moslems hold memorial services on the fortieth day after death. Annual anniversary services are also very common. Grieving and mourning are expected to be lengthy, often lasting several months after the death, but the dead person is usually not openly discussed for fear of upsetting close family members. Women wear black—often for months after the death—and men generally wear black ties at the funeral and memorial services. Prayers and religious chants for the deceased's soul are common practice.

Breaking the news of death to children is done gradually and tactfully. By the same token, close family members not present at the time of death are presented with the bad news gradually, often in stages. Communication of a grave diagnosis to the patient is also done in stages and with utmost tact. Iranian families feel that much harm can come from bluntly confronting the patient with a poor prognosis (Lipson and Meleis 1983). Iranians often complain that doctors in the West are insensitive to this issue and condemn the physician's directness in presenting the bad news. Canadian physicians may call in a single family member, preferably a male, to reveal the diagnosis to him tactfully and gradually.

NUTRITION AND FOOD

Iranians eat well and plentifully since food is the major medium for socializing. Family members eat together and mealtimes are for enjoying one another's company. In Iran, lunch used to be the most elaborate meal of the day, usually followed by a siesta. Since living conditions in Canada do not allow heavy and elaborate lunches, dinner has replaced lunch as the main meal of the day. Iranians sit at table and use cutlery for eating.

A staple in Iran is rice and Iranians boast about their many rich and lovely rice dishes and spend much time preparing them. Meat is an essential part of most Persian dishes; lamb, veal, beef, and chicken are the most popular. Fish is eaten in moderation, but other seafood like crab, lobster, and oysters is not commonly eaten. The consumption of pork is forbidden by Islam, as well as Judaism, and Iranians have generally not developed a taste for it. Oily food is preferred and animal fat remains popular. The use of different herbs is very common, but spices are employed in moderation (with the exception of saffron). Persian food is not hot or spicy. Iranians in Canada have maintained their traditional diet and continue to enjoy their home-made dishes. The consumption of junk food has, however, increased among children. Sugar consumption is rather high among Persians, which may account for early tooth decay in children.

OTHER IRANIANS IN CANADA

Some Canadian cities have attracted small Iranian populations of a sort that has not been discussed above. These are Iranian students who are sojourners in Canada and will return to Iran upon completion of degrees. This group is rather small and its members have a stronger attachment to the more traditional lifestyle of the homeland. For example, females in this group generally wear the Islamic "Hijab" or head and body cover and adhere strictly to Islamic laws. Some female patients from this group may insist on being seen by female physicians.

Similar to this group, in terms of religious practices, are other more devout Iranian Moslems, such as the Mujjahedin. These people have been victims of the present Iranian regime's persecutions for several years and have sought refuge in this country. Compared to the majority of Iranians in Canada, these groups have some fundamental differences, such as style of dress (particularly for women), strict adherence to religious practices (Islamic), and political ideology.

There is considerable variation in all the Iranian groups that have been described. The professional must find ways of learning about each client in order to understand how best to help that person and to avoid the hazards of generalizing and stereotyping.

FURTHER READING

Arasteh, A.R. *Man and Society in Iran*. Leiden, The Netherlands: Brill 1964

Bonine, M.E. and K. Keddie. *Continuity and Change in Modern Iran*. Albany: State University of New York Press 1981

Graham, R. *Iran: The Illusion of Power*. London: Croom Helm 1978

Haeri, S. "Women, Law and Social Change in Iran," in *Women in Contemporary Moslem Societies*. ed. J.I. Smith. NJ: Associated University Press 1980

Jalali, B. "Iranian Families," in *Ethnicity and Family Therapy*, eds. M. McGoldrick, J.K. Pearce, and J. Giordano. New York: Guilford Press 1982

Lipson, J.G. and A.I. Meleis. "Issues in Health Care of Middle Eastern Patients in Cross-cultural Medicine," *Journal of Western Medicine*, Vol. 139, No. 6 (1983): 854–61

Nyrop, R.F. *Iran: A Country Study*. Washington, DC: American University Press 1978

Zonis, M. *The Political Elite of Iran*. Princeton, NJ: Princeton University Press 1976

CONTRIBUTORS

P. Boustani (Physician, Vancouver)
Tali Conine (UBC)
Carol Herbert (Physician, UBC)
F. Mirhady (Physician, Vancouver)
K. Mirhady (Physician, Vancouver)
G. Partovi (Vancouver)
P. Partovi (Vancouver)
A. Raseky (Physician, Vancouver)

CHAPTER SIX

The Japanese

Teruko Okabe, Kazuko Takahashi, and Elizabeth Richardson

Japan extends 3,000 kilometres north to south in a crescent and is made up of four main islands: Hokkaido, Honshu, Shikoku, and Kyushu. The land area is about two-fifths the size of British Columbia; but the population is 121 million, five times that of Canada.

Most of Japan enjoys a temperate, oceanic climate with four distinct seasons. All areas, except the northernmost island of Hokkaido, have a hot, humid, rainy season (baiu) that lasts from early June to mid-July. Between August and October, the southwestern part of the archipelago is often hit by typhoons.

Japan's population is concentrated along the Pacific seaboard where the transportation and industrial facilities are most highly developed. Industrialization has been accompanied by a population shift towards the large cities and a decline in the agricultural areas.

Economic development since the Second World War can be divided into three periods: first, the recovery period during which Japan rebuilt its economy to the prewar level; second, a period of rapid growth; and third, a recent period of transition to a welfare-oriented economy with a stable growth rate.

Japan is a constitutional monarchy with a hereditary emperor and a parliamentary system of government. The emperor is ceremonial head of state and has little governmental power.

MIGRATION

The first Japanese immigrants to Canada arrived in British Columbia in the late nineteenth century; from 1896, a small number of farmers and fishermen left the overcrowded conditions of Japan annually in search of adventure and economic improvement. Until 1907, most newcomers to Canada were single men and many stayed only a few years, returning to Japan or migrating to the United States. Like the Chinese and South Asians, they experienced extreme ethnic discrimination and after an anti-Asian riot in 1907, the Canadian and Japanese governments agreed to regulate and restrict immigration to Canada. Wives and children, however, were allowed to join husbands and fathers already in Canada. Because of these restrictive immigration laws, there was virtually no immigration from Japan to Canada from the mid-1920s until the mid-1960s. Changes in Canadian immigration regulations in the latter period allowed the entry of many independent immigrants. In recent years, numbers have been low relative to many other immigrant groups, averaging roughly 400 to 500 annually since 1980. At present, the number of people of Japanese ancestry living in Canada is estimated to be over 50,000. Roughly 30 per cent live in British Columbia, with another 20 per cent in Ontario. The remainder are scattered across Canada, mostly in Alberta and Quebec. Most postwar immigrants have settled in urban areas.

Japanese Canadians may be divided into several groups. First generation immigrants who came to Canada prior to the Second World War are referred to as Issei. Most are now in their seventies and eighties. Reasons for migration included the desire for an increased standard of living and earnings, new cultural experiences, and to escape the restrictions of Japanese society. The majority of Nisei, or second generation Japanese Canadians, were born in Canada after 1910, mostly between 1920 and 1940. Kika Nisei refers to second generation Japanese who were born in Canada, educated in Japan, and then returned to Canada. The most recent immigrants, those who have come to Canada since the 1960s, are referred to as Shin-ijyusha. Like the Issei, they have come to Canada to find freedom, both social and economic. For many, migration represents a break away from lifetime employment with the same company, typical of Japan, and an opportunity to start new business enterprises and increase earnings. Finally, there are a significant number of temporary residents from Japan, mainly employees of Japanese companies, who are in Canada with their families on a short-term basis, generally a few years.

The information in this chapter focuses primarily on postwar immigrants who by virtue of being newcomers may experience most difficulty with the Canadian health care system because of differences in cultural belief and practice. These differences may exist in lesser degree for Issei and elderly Nisei and may therefore be relevant to their encounters with health care professionals as well. Younger generations of Japanese Canadians are unlikely to differ from other Canadians in their attitudes and behaviour regarding health care; most of what we present here does not apply to them.

In all ethnic groups, traditional beliefs, values, and customs may be retained in varying degrees by different individuals. Acculturation does not necessarily correlate with length of residence in Canada, and integration in one area does not imply a rejection of all traditional ways. For example, a second generation Japanese Canadian may be linguistically integrated but quite traditional in other aspects of behaviour. Apparently highly Westernized individuals may resort to traditional practices in times of illness, such as avoiding bathing, without being consciously aware that this behaviour is traditional. The extent of intra-ethnic diversity precludes generalized assumptions about people's beliefs and responses to different circumstances but, rather, necessitates assessment on an individual basis.

SOCIO-ECONOMIC BACKGROUND

For the most part, the Issei came from rural areas of Japan and generally did not have a high level of education. After coming to Canada, they had little time to learn English because they worked long hours to earn a living. They found employment in fishing, coal mining, and lumbering. The Nisei, or second generation, were educated within the Canadian school system and generally attained a higher level of education than their parents. The majority learned to speak English fluently and were able to act as interpreters for their parents. Most were sent to Japanese language schools, but many learned Japanese only incidentally.

In 1942, during the Second World War, men, women, and children of Japanese ancestry were removed from the Pacific coast of Canada. By far the majority were Canadian citizens. Men were separated from their families and sent to work camps. This disruption of the traditionally strong family unit, where the father and older sons had dominant positions, caused great anxiety and anguish. Homes, property, and livelihoods were lost without compensation. In 1945, the government issued an ultimatum whereby people had to choose between resettling east of the Rockies or applying for repatriation to Japan. It was not until 1949, four years after the war had ended, that Japanese Canadians were granted the right to vote and allowed to return to the BC coast.

Most postwar Japanese immigrants are from middle-class backgrounds with university education. They tend to be relatively young, independent, and confident. Most are involved in business in Canada. They come with a knowledge of English since it is part of the high school curriculum in Japan, and they are able to increase their fluency through night school, exposure on the job, from radio and television and by associating with other Canadians. Some immigrant women find employment outside the home and the type of work is usually dependent on their level of English. Typical occupations include hostesses in Japanese restaurants, tour guides, office workers in Japanese companies, factory workers, clerks, and employees in small businesses such as gardening or dry cleaning.

RELIGION

The principal religions in Japan are Shintoism, Buddhism, and Christianity. Most people in Japan are tolerant of religious beliefs and do not regard simultaneous involvement in several religions as being incongruous. For the most part in Japan, birth and marriage ceremonies are Shinto, and funerals are Buddhist.

The majority of Japanese immigrants to Canada are from the Buddhist-Shinto traditions, while the remainder are Christians. The first Buddhist temple was established in Vancouver in 1905. Services became social occasions as well as religious events, and provided respite from hard labour and loneliness for the predominantly male Japanese community. Buddhist temples, or churches as they came to be called, formed an important part of the social network of the local Japanese community, much like that of the Christian parish. They continue to function as a resource for newcomers from Japan. Many Japanese who came to Canada as Buddhists in the early part of this century converted to Christianity shortly thereafter.

As with the general Canadian population, only a small percentage of Japanese Canadians actively practice any religion.

Shintoism

Shinto or the "Way of the Gods" is the indigenous religion of Japan. It is polytheistic and Shinto gods or kami are worshipped at shrines. All natural objects and phenomena were considered to have kami, so that the gods of Shinto became innumerable.

Shintoism is largely concerned with obtaining the blessing of the gods for future events. Ceremonies are held to bless babies, children, weddings, and the start of new enterprises. Talismans (omamori), which can be purchased at Shinto shrines in Japan, serve a variety of health-related functions, such as the delivery of a healthy baby, speedy recovery from illness, successful surgery, and so on.

There are no Shinto shrines in Canada.

Buddhism

Buddhism reached Japan in the sixth century via China and Korea. It holds that the ultimate state is one of self-enlightenment which is attained by waking to the truth. There is no god in Buddhism; the emphasis is on ridding oneself of hate and jealousy through infinite love. Fanaticism is rejected and tolerance is desired.

Buddhism is a major presence in the life of people in Japan. Even if they are non-believers, they go to temples, are buried according to Buddhist rites and, after death, are given posthumous Buddhist names. Traditionally, a family altar is maintained in the household's place of honour. In it are kept the names of deceased family members. Regular ceremonies honour these ancestors. During the annual O-bon season (July or August), it is believed that the souls of the deceased return to visit. In Japan, people return to their traditional family homes at this time.

Buddhism has exerted a tremendous influence on every aspect of traditional Japanese culture, including art, literature, and architecture, as well as on the morals and modes of thought of the people.

FAMILY STRUCTURE

Traditionally, the Japanese lived together as extended families and still do in rural areas. Now, however, urban apartment dwelling in Japan emphasizes the nuclear family, and some Japanese express no desire for the elderly to live with them.

The husband's role is to work diligently at his job and to provide for the family. The wife is to respect, honour, and care for him. She is responsible for raising the children and managing the household. All the responsibility for child-rearing is hers including education and care during illness. However, in some matters, other family members are consulted before a decision is made. In making a health-related decision, for example whether to take a child to the doctor, weight is given to the opinion of family elders and the final decision is the husband's. Parents are devoted to meeting the physical and emotional needs of the children, and children are obliged to respect, honour, and obey parents. The mother-in-law may assume responsibility for ensuring that her daughter-in-law performs all her household and child-rearing duties properly.

A woman has an important role in the care of ill family members. It is her responsibility to attend to not only her children, but also her husband, her parents, and sometimes, her husband's parents. Her role in health care is not limited to times of illness, but is also preventive. She is responsible for the maintenance of her family's good health through diet and close attention to body states and functions. Although a woman nurtures her husband and children through illness, when she herself becomes more than mildly sick, she typically relies on her own mother's assistance as the husband's traditional role does not include care of his wife. In Canada, severe illness may cause additional stress for the woman who does not have her mother at hand to support her.

In Japan, women are brought up to marry and have children, so that in most cases, employment is considered temporary with relatively low status and low pay. In the past, most women had limited elementary school education, but now the majority attain junior college level before marrying or joining the work-force. Most Issei married in their early twenties but in modern Japan, most women marry by their late twenties or early thirties. In Japan, a woman is considered "old" in her late forties, when her children are no longer a responsibility or when they leave home. At this point she may take up hobbies or attend classes in the community to fill the gap created by her children's absence. It is a difficult period for women as they have devoted so much of their lives to their children.

The Japanese family has the duty and obligation to care for all its members, young and old, to take an active part in finding suitable partners for the children, and to educate and teach the children proper conduct. Family members are expected to stand together when dealing with outsiders. Within the family, the moods and feelings of others are highly respected, so that much interaction is indirect and non-verbal. Family wishes and appropriate conduct take precedence over individual desires. Respect is given to the wage-earner, to men, and to the elderly. Within the family hierarchy, the father has the most authority, then the grandfather, eldest son, mother, and daughter.

Conformity to rules of conduct and etiquette is an important aspect of Japanese culture, and family problems tend to be hidden from outsiders as they are felt they bring shame on the whole family. Examples of such problems include loss of work, mental illness, pregnancy out of wedlock, breaking the law, and dropping out of school. Financial problems and drinking may lead to aggression, for example, beating the wife or children. However, it is important to the family that outsiders remain unaware and uninvolved in these difficulties. Problem solving is dealt with first by the family itself. If this is unsuccessful, the family may seek an arbitrator, someone discreet whom the family respects, to assist without causing the family loss of face. It is very unlikely that the person chosen for this role will be a professional or stranger.

Traditionally, the elderly are revered and respected, and typically, the eldest son is responsible for his ageing parents. In Canada, however, the first born generally takes the initiative, or an unmarried daughter may assume responsibility.

In Japan, men retire between the ages of fifty-five and sixty-five. However, following retirement, many look for another job and work until seventy or seventy-five. To have some type of employment is considered very important, and for many, retirement connotes boredom and meaninglessness. Elderly women often assist in the care of grandchildren.

Many Issei did not achieve a high degree of integration into mainstream Canadian society. Whether they wanted to or not, they were prevented from doing so by social and legal discrimination. They maintained traditional Japanese values: strong ties to the family unit; respect for and obedience to elders; a dominant position for the father and an inferior position for women and children; and emphasis on thrift and hard work. It was economically necessary for most women to work outside the home. Many Issei have retained basic customs such as Japanese foods and traditional medicines. For many, the inability to communicate fluently in English persists as a problem, and many feel unhappy that the traditional values of loyalty, honour, and obligation are not upheld by the younger generations in Canada.

New immigrants to Canada often suffer stress due to differences in language and custom. Conflicts can occur when women attempt to maintain the traditional role of wife and mother while holding down full-time work outside the home. Those who are not employed may feel a loss in status as the housewife's role in Canada does not enjoy the high esteem that it does in Japan. Contact with non-Japanese women can encourage greater independence; for example a baby-sitter may be hired so that a wife can go out to dinner with her husband. If a man comes to Canada with fluent English or acquires it quickly, he retains his role of authority within the family. If, however, he has to rely on his children to translate, there is a reversal of dependence which may weaken his position. His authority may also be undermined by his wife becoming more independent.

MARRIAGE

Intermarriage with non-Japanese Canadians was very rare among Issei and Nisei. It has become common, however, for the third generation. Among post-Second World War immigrants, men tend to look for wives back in Japan where they are likely to find more traditional women, while young women often find marriage partners here in Canada. These may be either non-Japanese Canadians or members of the postwar Japanese immigrant community.

CHILD-REARING

The mother, or sometimes a female relative, takes care of the children, and child-rearing is a highly valued occupation in Japan. The mother is responsible for her children's education, for arranging tutoring, attending parent-teacher conferences, and so on. In Canada, fathers have more time to spend with their families because working hours are shorter, but they may be reluctant to become involved in school activities which they still believe to be the woman's role.

Babies are encouraged to be passive, and crying is discouraged out of deference to neighbours. This is because people in Japan live in small houses closely crowded together. Also, some may believe that keeping quiet is better for the child's health. Children are breast-fed until about one year of age. Toilet-training begins at seven to ten months by placing the child over the toilet, but there is no insistence that the child must succeed.

Generally, parents are very permissive with young children up to the age of about six or seven. Once they start school, discipline is increased. Tidiness and good manners are encouraged in the young child. Discipline involves the mother using consistency and teaching consideration for others. Instruction tends to be by example rather than verbal, as it is believed that children learn best by imitation. Light spanking is not uncommon, and punishment is exercised by threatening the child with abandonment or exclusion from the family, or by means of embarrassment or shame.

Children are taught to respect elders and those in authority; to distinguish between relatives and close friends (insiders) and others (outsiders); to develop giri or social sensitivity to the needs of others (parents, family, community); and to be modest and considerate. Children also learn that it is appropriate and acceptable to depend on others and to ask for favours (amaeru). Initially this dependence is on the mother and later is transferred to the group. Another important notion taught to children is that of gaman or the need to be stoical, to endure adversity patiently and without complaint.

In Japan, teenagers are expected to be diligent in their school work and generally do not have many responsibilities. There is a strong emphasis on achievement and school work takes priority over peer relationship. Part-time jobs are encouraged as long as studies are not compromised. Compared to those in North America, teenagers in Japan may appear immature and sheltered, as independence is discouraged. Teenage girls are not permitted to wear cosmetics or pierced earrings, and dating is disapproved of. Recent immigrants to Canada may be concerned about allowing teenage children to date, especially while they are still in high school.

NAMES

Customarily, the family name comes first and the given name second. Adults generally call each other by their family or surname and add the suffix san, meaning "Mr.," "Mrs.," or "Miss." An example is Tanaka san. Adults call children by their first names, adding kun for boys and chan mainly for girls. Children do not call older siblings by their first names, but use special terms meaning older brother and older sister. Women typically change their surnames when they marry, although recently in Japan some have chosen to keep their own names. This is, however, still considered to be very modern and unconventional.

GESTURES AND BODY LANGUAGE

Bowing indicates respect and is used for greeting or taking leave of others. The depth of the bow is generally a measure of the rank or status of the recipient. Handshakes are not common but are acceptable with Westerners.

Avoidance of eye contact traditionally denotes respect. However, most recognize and accept that eye contact is a feature of Western communication. In conversation, head nodding indicates attentiveness and understanding but not necessarily agreement. Similarly the statement, "I understand," means "I understand what you are saying" but does not always imply agreement or compliance. The physical expression of affection is open towards children, but occurs only discreetly or in private between spouses. Smiles may reflect a variety of emotions from joy to confusion, embarrassment, or politeness. Women especially, are acutely aware of and sensitive to non-verbal reactions, for example, facial expressions indicating hesitancy. They are quick to adjust so as to restore the comfort of the other person.

CONFLICT AND COMMUNICATION

From childhood, the expression of strong emotions, especially anger, is discouraged. Interpersonal harmony and co-operation are valued highly. Indirectness is used when revealing moods and feelings, and conflict and confrontation are avoided. Thus, agreement may be outwardly simulated in an attempt to maintain harmony. In such instances, a person may express disagreement indirectly by looking doubtful or remaining silent. Outside the family, conflict resolution and negotiation is occasionally accomplished by using a mediator (a priest, or respected friend) to assist in the process. When resolution is not achieved, indirect modes of aggression may occur, for example, gossip or avoidance.

SLEEPING PRACTICES

The preference in Japan is for more crowded and intimate sleeping arrangements over isolation in separate rooms; sleeping alone is considered pitiful and lonely. Children up to the age of five may share a bed mat (futon) with a parent or grandparent. The sharing of a room by pre-teenage siblings of both sexes is not uncommon. In Canada, Japanese families adopt Western-style beds and separate rooms for children.

CLOTHING

In Japan, people wear Western clothing in their everyday life, but traditional clothing is still popular as formal attire, for example, at weddings. Shoes should be removed when entering a home and slippers are worn indoors. In Canada, many Issei and postwar immigrants continue this custom.

SHOPPING

In Japan, women usually shop locally as everything is available in the neighbourhood. In Canada specialty shops dealing in Japanese items are generally located in downtown areas so that if women do not drive, they may have to rely on husbands for transportation.

UNLUCKY NUMBERS AND AGES

The numbers four, nine and thirteen are considered unlucky. The word "four" in Japanese is shi, which also means "death"; the character for "nine" is associated with a word meaning "suffering." Certain ages are believed to be potentially dangerous; these are nineteen, thirty-three and thirty-seven for women, and twenty-five, forty-two, and sixty-one for men.

RECREATION AND LEISURE

In Japan, watching television and reading are typical family leisure activities. Traditional sports (sumo wrestling, judo, karate, aikido) as well as modern ones (baseball, tennis, golf, swimming) are enjoyed. Calligraphy, flower arranging, bonsai, tea ceremonies, cooking, and sewing are common leisure activities for women. Sightseeing, locally and abroad, is popular.

In Japan, a woman is generally not expected to have much leisure time while she is rearing children. Men are expected to relax after work, for example by watching television at home, or eating and drinking with friends at a restaurant or bar. During the week, men who are white-collar workers often only come home to sleep; they work long hours and are expected to socialize with co-workers afterwards.

For the most part, dropping in unannounced is considered rude, and a home visit should be accompanied by a gift for the hostess. Guests are treated well, and typically tea is served with fruit and sweets.

In Canada, Issei seldom mix socially with non-Japanese in leisure activities. Nisei, or the second generation , mix well in sports and some social activities, while later generations have little sense of being different or separate from other Canadians.

FESTIVALS AND HOLIDAYS

There are many festivals celebrated throughout Japan. New Year is the main holiday season and many people return to their family homes at this time. People also return home during the summer holiday season of O-bon in order to visit the graves of their ancestors. There are special holidays to celebrate children, adulthood, and the aged.

In many Canadian urban centres the Japanese community holds a festival at O-bon season. It is a social gathering with food and dancing.

HEALTH CARE BELIEFS AND PRACTICES

The health care beliefs and practices of contemporary Japan derive from three main sources: the indigenous Shinto belief system, kanpo or the medical tradition brought to Japan from China in the sixth century, and the Western biomedical system.

Shinto Health Care Tradition

Early beliefs in Japan were that illness was caused by evil spirits or by exposure to polluting sources, such as blood, sick people, and dead bodies. Treatment involved purification rituals like hot spring baths and herbal infusions.

Kanpo or Traditional Japanese Medicine of Chinese Origin

This system is based on a belief that a person has the responsibility to take care of his health through careful attention to diet, sleep, exercise, and interpersonal relationships, since illness can result from an imbalance in these areas. There is also a belief that the universe, both physical and social, exists in a dynamic state of balance between two polar forces: yin and yang. Yin represents what is female, negative, dark, cold, and empty, while yang contains what is male, positive, light, warm, and full. Everything, including parts of the body, symptoms, and diseases, is ascribed yin and yang qualities. Body organs are believed to have specific relationships to one another, so that, for example, if the lungs are weak, the kidneys will show a weakness also.

The abdomen (hara), referring to stomach and intestines, is important in the traditional view of health and illness. There tends to be a greater fear about diseases of the stomach than other illnesses, as problems with the stomach are thought to affect the balance of the whole bodily system. Traditionally, a cloth was wrapped around the abdomen for protection (haramaki), and this practice is continued today in Japan, especially in the case of children, the aged, and pregnant women.

Also stemming from the classical Chinese medical tradition is the belief that man is affected by the natural environment so that attention is paid to the effect of climatic changes on the body. Neither the parts of the body, nor the whole person, function in isolation. Rather, they are parts of a dynamic, interdependent system.

A further belief is in the existence of a series of pressure points on the surface of the body. The stimulation of one point exerts an effect on another part of the body. Pathways which connect these points and allow for the transmission of energy are called meridians.

Treatment in traditional medicine is aimed at restoring bodily balance and harmony. The primary methods are herbal medicine, acupuncture, and moxibustion (the burning of small balls of moxa or dried mugwort on appropriate pressure points). Therapeutic massage techniques (shiatsu) are also used for muscle or joint problems, as well as general body weakness and fatigue. Traditionally, the pressure point system was used in shiatsu, but there are now different schools, some of which have incorporated chiropractic techniques. Diet is an important aspect of treatment, and corrective diets may be based on the classical concept of yin and yang foods. No synthetic drugs are used and surgery is not a part of this medical tradition, as it is believed to upset the bodily imbalance further. Treatment should be mild and is simply intended to boost the innate potential of the body to heal itself, a process which is slow and gradual. Attention is paid to mild symptoms as it is believed that ignoring them will lead to a worsening of the condition, which will then require lengthier treatment. In Japan, people generally turn to traditional medicine for chronic and degenerative illnesses, while help is sought from Western biomedicine for acute ones. For the most part, women are more familiar with traditional medicine than men.

In Japan, medicines are made from dried herbs, most of which are imported from China and are therefore expensive. The herbs are boiled and strained to make a bitter tasting liquid. Herbal medicines are believed to work gradually over a period of time, and small, mild and frequent doses are believed to be more beneficial than larger and stronger doses that are taken less often. In Japan, herbal medications are either prescribed and sold by doctors practising traditional medicine or purchased prepackaged at pharmacies. Their use has become more common in recent years as concern over the side effects of synthetic drugs has increased.

Both acupuncture and moxibustion use the meridian and pressure point systems. In the case of acupuncture, needles are inserted into the body at appropriate points. With moxibustion, heat is the source of stimulation, and small balls of ignited moxa or mugwort are left on the skin until it becomes hot. In some methods, another substance, for example, ginger, is placed between the moxa and the skin for protection. In others, the moxa is placed directly on the skin causing blisters and scarring. Acupuncture and moxibustion are used most often to treat muscular and skeletal problems. In Japan, both are practised by licensed paramedics, although moxibustion is also commonly used by people themselves at home to treat minor symptoms.

The involvement and co-operation of the patient and his family in the treatment process is considered an important part of therapy, and traditional practitioners spend time developing trust and rapport with patients.

Western Biomedical System in Japan

Biomedical health care facilities in Japan are excellent. There are large public hospitals as well as many small private hospitals and clinics which are owned and operated by doctors. Medical facilities are accessible to the neighbourhood, even in rural areas.

Virtually all Japanese are covered by health insurance either through the national government program or through their employers. The coverage is extensive and includes dental care as well as drugs, which are dispensed by physicians themselves. Neither prenatal examinations nor delivery are covered and must be paid for privately.

The influence of traditional medicine may be seen in the practice of biomedicine in Japan. Patients are encouraged to consult physicians for mild symptoms and conditions, for example, coughs, colds, or general feelings of fatigue. People are very sensitive to the possible side effects of drugs which tend to be less potent than those prescribed in North America, and are taken more frequently. After a patient has consulted a doctor about a complaint, he or she is asked to return for frequent check-ups, sometimes daily, when medication may be reviewed and reissued. In general, patients expect to receive some medication or treatment when they visit a doctor. Sometimes a family member will remain with a patient during an examination and occasionally, when a patient is unable to keep an appointment, a relative or close friend will attend in order to report on the patient's progress or receive medication or test results.

PREVALENCE OF DISEASE IN JAPAN

General health standards in Japan are very high. Infant mortality is low and the life expectancy in 1985 was seventy-five years for males and eighty years for females. The major causes of death are cardiac disease, cerebral haemorrhage, and cancer, the most common form being stomach cancer.

RELATIONSHIP BETWEEN DOCTOR AND PATIENT

Doctors enjoy very high status in Japanese society. Patients defer to them and will agree to everything said. At a medical consultation, a patient expects to have a thorough examination, to be asked about subtle body changes, and at the conclusion, to receive medication, and an explanation of the condition or illness.

Generally in Japan, doctors do not inform patients of a diagnosis of cancer, except in cases where there is a high probability of successful treatment. As cancer is popularly believed to lead to inevitable death, informing the patient is held to be too depressing and anxiety inducing and to lead to a worsening of the patient's condition. As a rule, the family is informed and they decide whether or not to tell the patient.

In Canada, finding a Japanese-speaking doctor is a high priority for Issei and postwar immigrants. Patients tend to be reluctant to discuss family or social problems with non-Japanese physicians, feeling that they do not understand the cultural context. Seeing a specialist in Japan does not require referral and many find the Canadian system inconvenient and a waste of time. Women tend to prefer female obstetricians and gynaecologists. In general, people find the Canadian patient-physician relationship more friendly and familiar than in Japan where it tends to be distant and formal.

In Japan, health care professionals who are not doctors have lower status. The function of nurses tends to be more like that of receptionists or secretaries. In Canada, patients accept treatment from a nurse provided that it has been authorized by the doctor.

MEDICATION AND TREATMENT

Japanese are concerned that Western drugs are strong and may cause side effects. However, compliance is usually good if regard for the doctor is high, that is, if the patient perceives the doctor as competent and appropriately formal in his conduct. Family members can influence compliance. For example, if an older member reacts to a prescribed medication, the daughter may discourage continued use by saying, "That medicine is too strong for you."

Some Issei and postwar immigrants use traditional medicines for chronic and mild conditions. Herbal medicines may be purchased in Vancouver's Chinatown and are considerably cheaper than in Japan. They are taken for allergies, stomach, and bowel problems, as well as for general health maintenance. A small number of these immigrants also use moxibustion as a home remedy for a variety of problems including back pain, shoulder stiffness, and general tension. Also, practitioners of acupuncture and shiatsu are consulted, although in Canada these specialists are not as prevalent, and may often be regarded as underqualified.

HOSPITALIZATION

The average length of stay in Japanese hospitals is longer than in Canada. This is due at least in part to a belief that during illness and recuperation people should receive extra care and attention as well as bed rest. Generally, family members play an active role in providing care during hospitalization, for example, by washing clothes, bringing meals, and staying with the patient for long periods.

In Japan, there is an expectation that, in addition to family, friends and co-workers will visit a hospitalized patient. Not visiting is likely to be interpreted as an expression of negative feelings. Visitors are expected to bring gifts, preferably of a perishable nature such as fruit or cut flowers, which symbolize the temporary nature of the illness and betoken a speedy recovery. Potted flowers, for example, would be inappropriate as they would suggest lengthy or permanent illness.

Generally, people prefer to use their own nightwear as hospital gowns are considered to be impersonal and to strengthen the sense of control over the situation. There may also be a dislike of wearing clothes that others have worn previously. Gowns with ties at the back are especially disliked as they compromise feelings of privacy.

In Canada, postwar immigrants and Issei generally are considered by health professionals to be ideal patients as they tend to be stoical, co-operative, grateful, uncomplaining, and unquestioning. Those who have difficulty with English may be afraid of not understanding the discussions, and recent immigrants may be unfamiliar with hospital routines or expectations. They may be embarrassed to ask for clarification and so agree to everything. Bathing can present a problem as many Japanese prefer a bath to a shower.

MENTAL HEALTH

Traditionally, mental illness is feared and stigmatized. When someone reaches marriageable age, for example, the family would discourage him or her from choosing a partner with a history of psychiatric treatment. There may be a tendency for families to hide members experiencing mental health problems and to be too ashamed to seek professional help. Thus treatment, especially hospitalization, is likely to be delayed until the family can no longer deal with the problem.

Generally, mental illness is expressed through somatization rather than by psychological complaints. Excessive sensitivity to the social and physical environment (shinkeishitsu) is a common culture-bound neurosis related to the inability to satisfy dependency needs (amaeru). Individuals suffering from this syndrome tend to be perfectionistic and highly self-conscious; they are also believed to be intelligent and creative. Physical symptoms include fatigue, sleeplessness, stomach-aches, and headaches. This neurosis is believed to stem from a childhood syndrome known as kan no mushi and is characterized by frequent crying, irritability, and temper tantrums. It is held to derive from over-indulgent and over-protective mothering, and to occur more commonly in boys than girls. Treatment for these neuroses is often sought in the realm of traditional medicine.

In Japan, young men may resort to suicide when the pressure to succeed is so great that failure represents a loss of face for the family. In the elderly, suicide may occur when role changes lead to feelings of unworthiness and alienation.

In Canada, depression is a common mental health problem among middle-aged housewives of the postwar immigrant community. Here, they lack the cultural support for the traditional role of wife and mother, particularly after their child-rearing years are over. If they have been influenced by the more liberated values of Canadian women, but are still part of a traditional, male-dominated marital relationship, they tend to experience conflict and depression. Husbands and children generally adapt more quickly to Canadian society as a result of exposure at work and school. Housewives, by contrast, are frequently left behind in linguistic and cultural isolation. These women rarely seek professional help of their own accord and most often are taken for it by friends or family members.

The forced removal and internment of Japanese Canadians during the Second World War is a potential source of mental health problems. There are many Japanese, particularly older people, who were relocated from West Coast areas to other provinces. Their homes, property, and businesses were expropriated, which generally prevented them from returning after they were legally allowed to, in 1949. Mental health problems sometimes followed, including suppression of anger, problems of identity, and depression. Many have been unable to obtain appropriate mental health treatment because of language and cultural barriers.

In Japan, talk is not considered appropriate treatment for mental health problems; it is simply a means to elicit information about physical symptoms. The treatment and elimination of "real" physical symptoms is thought to prevent the development of more complicated symptoms later on. The cultural values of interpersonal harmony and fulfilment of social roles, including service to the family, determine therapeutic goals for mental health problems. In general, the basic objective is to assist the individual to accept and adjust to his social environment, rather than to change it.

In western Canada, there are very few Japanese-speaking mental health professionals. Consequently, many people with minimal fluency in English end up with an English-speaking psychiatrist or mental health professional. The result is frustration in patients who have difficulty expressing themselves, and who may feel that the professional does not understand the cultural implications of their problem. Because of lack of experience and trust in mental health services here, many avoid seeking help until the problem becomes serious.

FAMILY PLANNING

Most couples start their families within the first two years of marriage, and the preference is for two or three children. Although traditionally boys were favoured as first born, many couples now have no special preference for the sex of offspring. Generally, the husband takes responsibility for contraception, using condoms or the rhythm method. Talking about sexual matters is embarrassing to both men and women, and sexual jokes are not considered in good taste, especially in the presence of unmarried women.

Although abortion is not sanctioned, since traditional Buddhist belief holds all life to be sacred, it is in fact quite common in Japan and accepted. Premarital sex is not condoned for women but is acceptable for men. If an unmarried woman becomes pregnant, she brings shame to the whole family. Thus in Japan, pregnancy is commonly hidden by sending the woman to stay with relatives until she has had an abortion. Illegitimate birth is strongly disapproved; the status of the child is low and the family loses face. In Japan, the family usually keeps the baby, but until recently in Canada, illegitimate children, especially those of mixed race, were given up for adoption.

PREGNANCY AND PRENATAL CARE

Customarily, a woman tells her husband and family as soon as she knows that she is pregnant. Pregnancy and birth are viewed as a happy and extremely valuable time by women, who are pampered and well taken care of during this period.

Eating well-balanced meals is an expectation during pregnancy. After the fifth month, salty and spicy foods are restricted while milk, seaweed, and soya beans are stressed. Fruit and vegetables are recommended to avoid constipation. In Canada, emphasis is placed on vitamins, dental care, regular medical visits, and prenatal classes. People with communicable diseases are avoided.

In Japan, visits may be made to a Shinto shrine to pray for a healthy baby. During the fifth month of pregnancy, on a day considered auspicious for easy delivery, a long white cotton sash is purchased at a temple or shrine. This is worn wrapped around the abdomen under the outer clothing for the remainder of the pregnancy and usually for about one month after delivery. It is believed to ward off illness by keeping the abdomen warm and is intended to prevent the foetus from moving around too much and from becoming too large, which would result in difficult delivery. It is also worn because it is considered to be comfortable. In Canada, many immigrant women continue this practice and are sent the sash by mothers or other relatives in Japan.

CHILDBIRTH

It is traditionally a mother's role to care for her daughter at the time of childbirth, and in Japan it is not uncommon for a woman to return to her family home, especially for the birth of the first child. For this reason, it is accepted that the doctor who sees a woman during her pregnancy is often not the one who delivers the baby. For subsequent births, the mother usually comes to her daughter's own home to help her.

In Japan, childbirth is usually at a neighbourhood hospital with a doctor and midwife attending. Generally the husband is not present at the birth. Gowns are not supplied by the hospital and women wear their own clothing in labour. The preferred position for childbirth is in bed with the head raised. Anaesthetics are available but decorum during painful bouts is considered important, so women appear stoical. Babies are taken to the nursery immediately after birth and given glucose water. Circumcision is not performed.

In Japan, pregnancy and childbirth belong exclusively to the realm of women. However, in the case of postwar immigrants to Canada, husbands, although perhaps embarrassed and uncomfortable, show interest in attending prenatal classes and in attending the birth, if only to interpret for their wives. Often the mother or mother-in-law is not here to provide the customary care and support.

POSTPARTUM PERIOD

It is traditional to present the infant's navel cord to the mother when she is discharged from hospital (heso-no-o). Preservative is sprinkled on the cord and it is placed in a wooden box which is tied with a ribbon. This custom continues in some, but not all, hospitals in Japan. However, this presents no real problem in Canada as women do not expect the practice to be honoured here.

In Canada, the postpartum period may be difficult for the woman who, in the absence of her mother or mother-in-law, is unable to receive the usual extra help and support. For the first month, a new mother is not expected to go out or do anything except breast-feed the baby. During this period, the family receives visitors, unless the baby is premature or abnormal, in which case people may be too embarrassed to visit.

In Japan, a newborn baby, especially a first born, is taken by parents and grandparents to a Shinto shrine for blessings and prayers for a long life. When a baby is born to Japanese immigrants in Canada, family members in Japan may visit a local shrine and send talismans commemorating the visit.

In Japan, weaning takes place later than in Canada, and breast-feeding to one year of age is not uncommon especially as most women are not employed outside the home. In Canada, where many Japanese women have to return to work, babies are weaned earlier, although generally breast-feeding is preferred to bottle-feeding.

Postpartum depression as such is not known, and as mentioned above, mental health problems in general tend to be hidden or ignored.

CHILDHOOD HEALTH AND ILLNESS

Common childhood diseases are colds, chest conditions, ear infections, and stomach-aches. There is a very old belief that leaving a crying child unattended is unhealthy as it may result in hernia or a protruding navel due to over-exertion. During mild illnesses, feeding, bathing, and massaging by the mother reinforce the bonds of family interdependency and are considered important in preventing more serious conditions. Home treatments include herbal remedies for colds and general malaise. The attitude towards vaccinations is positive since prevention of disease is welcomed. A sickly child arouses great concern because it requires extra care and because its condition may reflect negatively on the family.

DISABILITY AND CHRONIC DISEASE

Families are concerned about physically and mentally disabled members, but may also feel shame and embarrassment. They therefore may be reluctant to discuss problems or seek support and may tend to hide treatment.

Children under the age of fifteen who have chronic diseases, such as asthma, eczema, and nephrosis, are the responsibility of the mother. In general, compliance with treatment depends on the degree of satisfaction with the physician. A low rate of compliance may be due to poor explanation, wrong diagnosis, overprescription of medication, too many injections, or apparent lack of concern. Patients may be reticent to inform a physician about problems with treatment regimens, such as side-effects.

HYGIENE AND BATHING

Deriving from traditional Shinto notions of impurity and pollution, many aspects of the world such as physical space and the body are classified as clean, pure, and safe on the one hand, and as dirty, polluted, and contaminating on the other. The "outside" is associated with impurity and so a Japanese removes his shoes and washes his hands on returning home. Within the home, the toilet is considered the least clean area, and in Japan, is always separated from the bathing area. The lower body, from the waist down, is believed to be less clean than the upper half. This division may even be reflected, for example, in the separate laundering of clothes worn on the upper body from those worn on the lower half of the body. Because of a traditional belief in the contaminating qualities of blood, menstruating women may consider themselves unclean.

Shinto belief stresses the importance of expelling poisons from the body so that enemas, frequent bathing, and gargling are considered basic to good health. In Japan, people do not use baths simply to wash themselves; in fact, the actual washing and rinsing are done outside the tub. The bath itself is a long, leisurely soak in a deep tub full of very hot water. Family members use the same bath water in turn, and the tub is emptied after the last person has finished. Customarily, bathing is done at night. In Canada, a deep bath is preferred to a shower as the purpose is not only cleanliness but also relaxation.

Bathing is associated with good health, and is usually avoided during periods of illness, especially fevers or upper respiratory infections. Thus, resumption of bathing signals recovery. Women often avoid hot baths while menstruating.

DENTAL HEALTH

Until the 1950s, before dental insurance was generally available in Japan, people usually went to a dentist only when they had toothache. Even now, fillings tend to be favoured because of the expense of dentures and restorative work. Due to the poor state of dental hygiene and prevention in Japan, as well as the popularity of sweets, people tend to develop dental caries early. In Canada, Issei generally regard preventive dental care as unimportant.

FOOD AND NUTRITION

The traditional diet in Japan consists of white and brown rice, soybeans, fish, salted pickles, fermented soybean paste (miso), noodles, soybean curds (tofu), green onions, spinach, yam, Japanese radish, eggs, seaweed, bamboo, mushrooms, greens, grapes, oranges, and other fruits. This diet is low in fats but high in salt. A traditional breakfast is rice, fish, pickles, and soup although many now have toast and coffee. Typically, lunch and dinner include rice, fish, vegetables, and clear soup. Between meals, a variety of sweets is available. Many elderly people do not like beef or bread, although these foods are now very common in Japan.

After moving to Canada, Japanese immigrants tend to include more foods that are high in sugar and low in nutritional value in their diet. In the home, women are responsible for food preparation which is time-consuming as it requires a great deal of chopping. Eating utensils are chopsticks, and slurping while eating soup noodles is acceptable and indicates appreciativeness.

Egg in sake (Japanese wine) is eaten for head colds, and some people eat hot noodle soup to induce sweating in cases of mild fever. Hot, soup-like steamed rice (konji) is eaten for diarrhoea or when recovering from surgery or serious illness. Ginseng tea, garlic, garlic wine, green onion, mushrooms, and salted plums are taken to maintain good health and prevent illness. It is extremely difficult for people to give up soy sauce and salted pickles when a low salt diet is prescribed. They may complain that there is nothing left for them to eat, although a low salt soy sauce is now available on the market.

USE OF ALCOHOL AND TOBACCO

Drinking alcohol is more acceptable for men in Japan than it is in Canada. Moderate over-indulgence is tolerated by wives and others as normal for it is believed to relieve stress. While occasional drunkenness is not uncommon, alcoholism is extremely rare. Drinking is usually done at bars or in the home. Although women traditionally drank very little, this is less true of young women, especially in Canada.

Many men smoke cigarettes, but few women do.

CARE OF THE ELDERLY

There are relatively few elderly postwar immigrants compared to the Issei and elderly Nisei. Recent elderly immigrants generally join families who are already settled here. Occasionally, families are unable to adjust to this situation, or the aged parent becomes a burden and has to be placed in a nursing home. In these cases the elderly individual experiences extreme culture shock and social isolation due to complete unfamiliarity with the language, food, and culture.

Many Issei and elderly Nisei live independently in self-contained apartments, often in low income housing. Most have families, but prefer living independently to being a burden. Many live near other Issei and elderly Nisei who form their social network. They are consequently less isolated and lonely than if they were scattered in the suburban homes of their families.

Because of the history of social and governmental discrimination in Canada, many elderly Japanese Canadians fear and distrust any type of formal authority. This attitude creates problems in care facilities and hospitals and often results in a high degree of stress and anxiety. Differences in food and lack of fluency in English are also significant problems for those in institutions. Moreover, institutionalized elderly tend to be scattered in many different care facilities, further contributing to their loneliness and alienation.

Generally, families feel guilt and shame about placing aged parents in institutions, and some may wish to keep the fact hidden from friends. At the same time, both husband and wife are often employed and unable to provide the necessary care for a frail or disabled parent.

DEATH AND DYING

The Buddhist belief in reincarnation along with established com-

memorative rituals for the deceased provide comfort and reconcile-
ment. After death, a Buddhist is given a name (ho-myo) by a priest
attended by the family. A wake is held on the evening before the
funeral, which is by cremation. Additional services are held on the
seventh and forty-ninth days, and services for the happiness of the
dead are held on the first, second, sixth, and twelfth anniversaries. It
is believed that the recently deceased are contaminating, and that
funerals, memorial services, and associated rituals counteract the
essential pollution associated with death. For example, salt is
sprinkled over those returning home from a funeral as an act of
purification. Many families maintain an altar in their homes where
deceased members are made offerings at special celebrations.

Japanese Christians naturally have funeral services in that tradition.

It is considered preferable to die at home than in hospital, and in
cases of terminal illness in Japan, doctors may advise willing families
to take the patient home. However, this is the ideal, and many families feel unable to cope with a dying patient in the home. When
someone is dying, the family is responsible for contacting relatives
and friends who are expected to pay their last respects. The family
decides on the treatment of the body after death. Because of the
stigma associated with cancer, families are reluctant to acknowledge
it as the cause of death.

USE OF HEALTH AND SOCIAL SERVICES

Strongly affected by their experiences during the Second World War,
Issei and elderly Nisei are conservative in attitude and lifestyle. In
general, they do not trust professionals and do not welcome their
involvement. Postwar immigrants for the most part are receptive to
professional support.

DELIVERING CULTURALLY SENSITIVE HEALTH CARE

Postwar immigrants and Issei often do not understand English well,
even if they seem able to speak it. Writing down instructions is a
good way to confirm information as it will usually be checked by
other people at home. It is best to avoid confrontation as it causes
embarrassment and people are afraid of losing face. It is important
to be aware that sexual matters and family problems are difficult
areas to deal with because they are considered extremely private.

FURTHER READING

Lebra, Takie Sugiyama. *Japanese Patterns of Behavior*. Honolulu: University of Hawaii Press 1979

Lock, Margaret. "Japanese Responses to Social Change: Making the Strange Familiar," *The Western Journal of Medicine*, Vol. 139, No. 6 (1983): 25–30

—"Popular conceptions of Mental Health in Japan," in *Cultural Conceptions of Mental Health and Therapy*. eds. A.J. Marsella and G. White. Boston: Reidel 1982

Nakane, C. *Japanese Society*. Berkeley: University of California Press 1970

CONTRIBUTORS

Kouichi Asano (Physician, Vancouver)
Ruth Coles (Mount St. Joseph Hospital, Vancouver)
Diane Kage (AMSSA, Vancouver)
Tatsuo Kage (MOSAIC, Vancouver)
Rose Murakami (Health Sciences Hospital, UBC)
Reverend Gordon Nakayama (Vancouver)
Diane Nishii (Vancouver)
Sakuya Nishimura (Burnaby)
Fumitaka and Masako Noda (Physicians, Vancouver)
Ken Shikaze (Tonari Gumi, Vancouver)

CHAPTER SEVEN

The South Asians

Shashi Assanand, Maud Dias,
Elizabeth Richardson, and
Nancy Waxler-Morrison

Here we use the term "South Asian" to refer to people with cultural origins in the Indian subcontinent, which includes Pakistan, India, Sri Lanka, Bangladesh, and Nepal. Although most South Asians in Canada have come from those countries, people of South Asian cultural heritage have also immigrated to Canada from other parts of the world, including the South Pacific (Fiji) and East Africa. Thus the South Asians in Canada are far from being a homogeneous group and represent great social and cultural diversity. Further differences are introduced by variations in urban and rural background, and levels of education. All share a common British colonial heritage and those with an educated, urban background have prior knowledge of the English language and of many aspects of Western culture when they arrive in Canada. In contrast, South Asian immigrants from rural areas often find the cultural gap very wide.

Diversity in health beliefs, practices, and experiences, both at home and in Canada, mirrors the general cultural and social diversity among South Asians. It is impossible to document such diversity in detail here, for example, differences in childbirth customs between Fijian and Ugandan Asians, or the well-educated New Delhi Hindu's expectations of his or her physician as contrasted with those of a Sikh farmer from the Punjab. Instead, we present some of the more widely held South Asian beliefs, practices, and experiences and indicate, where possible, how these vary. While immigrants from Sri Lanka have cultural backgrounds and beliefs similar to many other South Asians, their experience of free Western-style medical services differentiates them from others. For that reason, Sri Lanka is not covered in this chapter. Instead, many of our examples are from India. The health professional will wish to understand these common patterns but must recognize that differences between South Asians are great, depending on country of origin, religious affiliation, class, and degree or urbanization.

SOUTH ASIANS IN CANADA

The first South Asian immigrants to Canada arrived in B.C. around 1900. The early immigrants were predominantly Sikh men from the Indian state of Punjab who came here to earn money. Most found work in the forest industry, particularly in the sawmills of Victoria, Vancouver, and New Westminster. In 1909, South Asian immigration was banned although the ban was modified in 1919 to allow wives and children to join husbands and fathers. Because of restrictions on immigration there were only about 6,000 South Asians in Canada by 1942.

The ban was lifted in 1947; South Asian immigration increased dramatically after 1961 and increased even more in the 1970s as a result of changes in immigration regulations. Until 1961, the majority of South Asian immigrants were Sikhs from rural areas in northern India who found employment as unskilled workers. However, changes in immigration regulations in the 1960s resulted in people coming from all parts of India and from Pakistan, mostly highly educated technicians and professionals. In the 1970s, there was significant migration from Fiji and East Africa. Unlike the majority of Sikhs, who are rural people, other South Asians have come mostly from urban settings. There are now approximately 300,000 South Asians living in Canada, mostly in urban centres. While the majority of these are first generation immigrants, there are many now who are Canadian-born.

Most South Asians have migrated to Canada to pursue economic and educational opportunities that are perceived to be better than those of their home countries. A relatively small number, mostly from Sri Lanka, have come as political refugees. Many who came with higher education experienced downward occupational mobility because of lack of Canadian training and experience. The majority of South Asians in Canada are employed in white-collar and skilled blue-collar jobs.

HOME COUNTRIES AND REASONS FOR MIGRATION

The majority of people with South Asian cultural backgrounds who have migrated to Canada have come from India, Pakistan, East Africa, and Fiji. While they all have many basic beliefs and practices in common other characteristics and experiences are peculiar to each home country. For that reason, it is important to know something about each country, especially the quality of life there and the conditions under which South Asians left home and moved to Canada.

India

After gaining independence from Great Britain in 1947, India's democratic government took on the enormous challenge of social and economic development in a country which displayed great diversity. The presence of jungles, a desert, plains, tropical lowlands, and high mountains suggests the variety of ways in which people in India live and work. There are eighteen recognized languages and several hundred dialects indicating considerable social diversity. Some people speak their own language plus Hindi, the official language, and 2 per cent speak English.

Until recently India experienced relatively slow economic progress, the fundamental problem being the rapidly growing population which needed food, clothing, shelter, and education. Since the early 1900s the Indian population has grown by several million a year and has now reached 790 million, the second largest in the world. Three-quarters of the population are farmers, and overcrowding and pressure on agricultural land have meant that many rural villagers have crowded into the cities looking for work. Industrial development since independence has placed India among the top twenty industrial nations in the world. Benefits of this development have been unevenly distributed so that a small urban elite enjoys a high standard of living, yet very large numbers of Indians live at or below subsistence level.

Recent statistics suggest improvements. Since 1950 life expectancy has risen from about thirty-two years to about fifty-three years. As a result of expanded education programs, about 36 per cent of all adults are now literate. Education for all between ages six and fourteen is legally required but many villages have no schools and no teachers. Moreover, even where they do exist, children of poor families often leave school to work on farms to supplement family income.

About 83 per cent of the Indian population is Hindu and 11 per cent is Muslim. Other small religious groups are Christians, Sikhs, Buddhists, and Jains. Conflict between Hindus and Muslims occurred when India and Pakistan separated in 1947 and has flared up between Sikhs and the central government since 1982 and more especially since 1984 when the government launched a military attack on the Sikh Golden Temple.

The Sikhs from northern India, particularly the Punjab, represent the largest group of migrants from India. Most have come to Canada through sponsorship by relatives who were already settled in the country. Many were farmers or landowners with relatively little formal education or English, although by the standards of India's villages, they were relatively well off. In Canada, they work in lumber mills, the construction industry, and as janitors, farm workers, and taxi drivers. Many have started their own businesses. The majority of women work outside the home as unskilled farm workers, janitors, and factory workers, and in restaurant kitchens and canneries. Educated, urban Sikhs are employed in a variety of professions and technical positions. The largest Sikh population is in B.C.'s Lower Mainland and in Victoria, Duncan, and Nanaimo. There are also sizeable communities in Edmonton, Calgary, Winnipeg, and Toronto.

The next largest group of immigrants from India are Hindi- and Punjabi-speakers from northern India who, for the most part, are Hindu. The majority of these immigrants were part of a large wave of South Asian professionals who came to Canada in the mid-1960s. In general, this group was highly educated and middle or upper class. Many came to Canada from the United States, where they had been attending university, and most were independent immigrants who did not have relatives to sponsor them.

Immigrants from south India form a much smaller group. Most are either Hindu or Christian. Many are trained teachers who accepted teaching positions in rural areas and others are health professionals, accountants, and engineers.

Pakistan and Bangladesh

Pakistan is a Muslim nation, about 97 per cent of the population practises Islam and 1.5 per cent is Christian. Most of the country has a dry climate with hot summers and cool winters. The economy is based largely on agriculture and herding, and about 75 per cent of the population lives in rural villages. Most city people are factory workers or shopkeepers with little education. However, the urban population also includes educated middle- and upper-class people who have adopted many Western styles and ideas. The official language is Urdu, although the majority speaks various dialects of Punjabi as a first language.

During the 1800s and early 1900s Britain ruled that part of the subcontinent which became Pakistan. At partition, Pakistan was created out of northwest and northeast India and called, respectively, West and East Pakistan. These two sections had little in common except religion and the tensions erupted in civil war in 1971 when East Pakistan declared itself the independent state of Bangladesh.

Of the relatively few Bangladeshi immigrants to Canada, recently averaging about seventy-five per year, most came after independence in 1971 and settled in Ontario. The majority are highly educated and have technical training and almost all are Sunni Muslims.

Most Pakistanis came to Canada after 1967 and the majority entered the country as independent, not sponsored immigrants. Most are highly educated, of upper- or middle-class background, and are proficient in English. About half are professionals including teachers, doctors, scientists, and university professors and originated in the urban centres of Pakistan. In general the group is young although recently a number of aged parents have joined their families. More than 85 per cent are Sunni Muslims. Of the recent immigrants from Pakistan, averaging about 800 per year, most have settled in urban areas in Ontario, Quebec, and Alberta.

East Africa

People of South Asian culture have come to Canada from three East African countries—Uganda, Kenya, and Tanzania. All three were British colonies until the post Second World War period; all have predominantly rural populations performing agricultural work. Black Africans compose the majority of the population in each country. While Swahili and other local languages were and are used in rural areas, English was commonly used in urban areas among middle-class people. Since independence from British rule (Uganda, 1962; Kenya, 1963; Tanzania, 1964) economic and political policies have changed, and unrest and conflict have been common, particularly in Uganda. These changes have directly affected the decisions of people of South Asian origin to leave.

From the late nineteenth century, many Indians emigrated to the British colonies in East Africa in search of better economic opportunities. For the most part they were traders and entrepreneurs and came to play a dominant role as middlemen in the colonial economies of Uganda, Kenya, and Tanzania. Most lived in urban areas and small towns.

Over the years the South Asians' economic success and prominence came to be resented by the indigenous African majority. Thus, as the East African countries became independent in the early 1960s, the position of South Asians deteriorated. In 1972 the Ugandan dictator, Idi Amin, ordered the expulsion of all South Asians from the country and 6,000 migrated to Canada as political refugees. About 30 per cent were professionals, and about 50 per cent had been in business. Most of the rest were skilled workers. South Asians left Kenya after independence when the government took over many farms and businesses owned by non-Africans. At the same time South Asians were leaving Tanzania. Many immigrated to Canada, some directly, others via Britain.

The majority of South Asian immigrants from East Africa are Ismailis, a branch of the Shia sect of Islam, although some are Hindus and Sunni Muslims. Many South Asians from East Africa are now involved in business enterprises while others are professionals in the medical, legal, and commercial fields. In western Canada, the largest population is in the Greater Vancouver area but many also live in Edmonton and Calgary.

Fiji

Fiji is a tropical, South Pacific country made up of more than 800 scattered islands. The economy is based on agriculture and tourism, and the main crops are sugar cane, coconuts, ginger, and tobacco. English is the official language while Fijian and Fiji-Hindi are the other main languages.

About 45 per cent of the population are native Fijians, of Melanesian and Polynesian descent, and approximately 50 per cent are of Indian descent. The remaining 5 per cent boast Chinese, European, and other ancestry. Indo-Fijians control much of Fiji's business and industry.

Fiji gained independence in 1970 after having been a British colony since 1874.

South Asian Fijians are for the most part descendants of indentured labourers who arrived from India before 1920 to work on the sugar plantations. Over the years they achieved prominence in retail trade and transportation. In the 1960s, a small number of South Asian Fijians entered Canada. Immigration increased significantly after Fiji became independent in 1970 as a result of racial conflict and increasing political and economic tension. However, political conflict between the South Asian majority and the minority Fijians erupted in 1987, which accelerated the migration of South Asians from Fiji to Canada. On average, about 500 people now migrate each year.

There are now about 14,000 South Asian Fijians in Canada. Roughly 75 per cent live in Vancouver and many of the remainder have settled in Alberta. Most are proficient in English as it is the language of instruction in the British-style education system in Fiji. Relatively few of the immigrants are professionals; the majority are skilled and semi-skilled workers. Most have been unable to find comparable employment here and have had to accept whatever jobs they could find typically in small manufacturing plants and in the service industry. The majority of South Asians from Fiji are Hindu; about 15 per cent are Muslim.

LANGUAGE

The languages most commonly spoken by South Asians in Canada are English, Punjabi, Hindi, Gujarati, and Urdu. Those immigrants with higher education are already proficient in English when they come to Canada, while immigrants from rural areas without much formal education may have little literacy in their first language and little or no knowledge of English. Among the latter, it is the men who tend to acquire English more quickly than the women and the elderly. This is because of the men's daily exposure to it in the work place and because English is necessary for job advancement. Some women are reluctant to learn English and tend to avoid formal language training, unless it is required for employment or citizenship. They also have difficulty in integrating full-time jobs with language classes. Many women cope by relying on their husbands or children.

RELIGION

The most common religious groups in the South Asian communities in Canada are the Hindus, Sikhs, and Muslims, although there are also some Jains and Christians.

Hinduism

Hinduism has no single founder but rather denotes a broad range of cultural patterns that include religious rituals, family and social relationships, and general attitudes towards life. These patterns are sanctioned by reference to sacred scriptures and a variety of deities.

A feature of Hinduism is its tolerance of diversity. An ancient religion, it constantly absorbed and reinterpreted the beliefs and practices of the peoples with whom it came into contact. There is thus widespread variation in, for example, food habits, styles of dress, and forms of worship.

There are, however, some fundamental notions common to Hindu culture. One is the concept of the unity of life; that all life is interdependent, both human and animal. Life is a continuous circle without beginning or end, so that death and birth are merely transformations of form. After death, the soul is reborn in another life form.

All actions have consequences which must return to the perpetrator. The fortunes of the soul in each rebirth are determined by behaviour in former lives. This is the law of karma whereby the present is affected by past action, and the future by present action. Another notion is that society is organized into a hierarchy of social classes called castes, into one of which each individual is born. Each caste has its own rules of behaviour which include social contacts with members of other castes. For example, inter-caste marriage seldom occurs. Each caste also has rules about who may cook the food its members eat. Most Hindus will eat food prepared by members of a higher caste; thus people of the highest caste may eat only food prepared by fellow members. While education and modern industrial life have weakened some caste barriers the prohibition on inter-caste marriage is still strong.

Most Hindu religious activity centres on the home, and may involve the family, an individual, or perhaps a few friends. Many rites mark important life cycle transitions. For example, traditionally, the birth ceremony takes place before the umbilical cord is cut, and about ten days later there is a naming rite. Among high-caste Brahmins, a rite is performed when a boy reaches puberty. At that time he is given a sacred thread which is tied across one shoulder and around his waist for the rest of his life.

In 1983, the Hindu Council of Canada was established to act as a central organization for Hindus.

Sikhism

A relatively new religion, Sikhism was founded in northern India at the end of the fifteenth century by Guru Nanak. He sought to combine Hindu and Muslim elements in a single religious creed. His teachings embodied belief in a single God and the equality of all people and he rejected the caste system. Sikhism includes Hindu concepts of reincarnation as well as karma. Unlike Hinduism, the representation of God in pictures, and the worship of idols are forbidden. Worship within the Sikh brotherhood, or community, is important. Guru Nanak was followed by nine gurus, or masters, the last of whom was Guru Gopind Singh. The writings of the early Gurus were compiled in the Sri Guru Granth Sahib, the Sikh sacred book.

No specific birth rites are prescribed although a newborn baby is taken to the temple to be named. The most important ceremony for a Sikh is that of baptism. Although there is no set age for this, it is believed that a person should be capable of assuming responsibility for his or her decisions before being baptized. Not all Sikhs, however, decide to be baptized.

Baptized Sikh men are enjoined to wear turbans and do not cut their hair or beards. They wear a comb, white undershorts symbolic of chastity and typical of soldiers, and a small, symbolic sword. In addition, baptized men and women do not smoke or drink alcohol. Most men and women, whether baptized or not, wear a steel bracelet on the right wrist. Some Sikhs are vegetarian but this is a matter of personal choice.

The Sikh temple is a meeting place where both religious and social activities are held. There is no "Sabbath day" for the Sikhs, and prayer ceremonies are held every day. However, to conform to Western work schedules in Canada, a weekly religious service is held from Friday morning through Sunday afternoon. During this time, male and female members participate in the reading of the Granth Sahib, members taking turns to read for two hours at a time until the entire scripture has been completed. People may attend the service at any time during the weekend, and at its conclusion, a vegetarian lunch, prepared by members of the temple, is served. There are Sikh temples in many cities in Canada as well as in small towns with substantial Sikh populations.

Islam

The word "Islam" literally means "submission" and a Muslim is one who submits to the will of God, rejects all other gods, and follows the teachings of the Koran, the holy book which records the will of God as revealed to the prophet, Muhammad (570–632 AD). The central belief of Islam is expressed in the phrase: "There is no god but God ["Allah" in Arabic] and Muhammad is his Prophet." This statement of faith is repeated on many ritual occasions. Islam imposes a code of ethical conduct encouraging generosity, fairness, honesty, and respect. Muslims are required to pray five times daily, facing the direction of Mecca, after a ritual washing and they should additionally attend a mosque to pray together on Friday. They are to abstain from food, drink, and sexual activity from dawn to dusk during the month of Ramadan, the ninth month of the lunar Muslim calendar. Since the months of the lunar calendar derive from the solar year, Ramadan falls at a somewhat different time each year. Adultery and gambling are forbidden as are the consumption of pork and alcohol. Other meat and chicken must be killed in a prescribed manner.

Shortly after the death of Muhammad, Muslims divided into two major sects over the issue of who should succeed the prophet as religious leader. These sects are known as Sunni and Shia. Ismailis are one of the Shia subsects and many Ismailis from Gujarat state in India emigrated to East Africa after the late nineteenth century.

FESTIVALS AND RELIGIOUS HOLIDAYS

Diwali or the Hindu "Festival of Lights" is celebrated in October or November to give thanks for prosperity.

Holi is a Hindu spring festival from northern India and is celebrated in February or March to mark the end of the cold weather. It is a day of fun when sweets and gifts are exchanged.

Baisakhi is the major festival of the Sikhs celebrated by worship and dance each 14 April.

Ramadan is sacred for Muslims as the month in which Muhammad received the first of his revelations from God and is observed by fasting during daylight hours. A festive day is celebrated at the end of the month when the fast is broken.

FAMILY STRUCTURE

In South Asian culture, the family is the most important social unit. It consists of not just the nuclear grouping of parents and children but also includes grandparents, brothers, sisters, and their families. Traditionally, the extended family lives together in one household so that, for example, in the grandfather's household, his unmarried daughters, all his sons, and their families live together.

The extended family provides the identity of the individual as well as economic and emotional security. Interdependence is valued highly and the lifestyle is collective rather than individualistic. Ideally, earnings are shared and the whole family prospers together.

In Canada, the South Asian extended family continues to be a close-knit, interdependent unit. In many cases, brothers and their families live together with their parents. Traditionally, parents do not live with a married daughter and her family. However, after immigrating to Canada, a daughter may sponsor her parents who then come to live in her household. Today many South Asians in

Canada live as nuclear units. Nevertheless, their sentiments and behaviour continue to be those of the extended family.

Earnings are often pooled in an extended family. In some families, income is given to the grandmother who is then responsible for the household finances and allocates money to the daughter-in-law to run the household. In other cases, the eldest son may manage the family's finances.

Most decisions are made by the head of the household who is usually the most established, financially secure male. On all important matters close relatives are consulted and their opinions are given considerable weight. Health care decisions, for example, when to consult a doctor about an ill child, are made by the senior members of the family. Care for ill family members is the responsibility of the wife or mother. In Canada, just as in her home country, she is likely to be assisted by grandparents or other relatives.

If the extended family unit is working together well, it is a highly supportive system. It is not necessary, for example, to find baby-sitters, as grandparents or other relatives are available. If a woman is sick, she is able to take a day off while someone else takes over the cooking, cleaning, and child care. However, if the family is dysfunctional, a woman may find difficulty in taking time off from household duties because of family censure.

Traditional South Asian culture is male-dominated and sex roles are well-defined. The man has the leadership role as head of the family, provider, and major decision-maker. The woman is in charge of nurturing and performing household duties. Her most important responsibility is to look after her family and her training is totally geared towards her role in the home. Traditionally, women did not work outside the home and they were therefore financially dependent on their husbands.

In traditional culture, a woman is seen as her husband's possession and she is taught to be submissive and to obey him. In spite of this asymmetry, women and girls nevertheless have high social and religious status. They are considered to bear the honour of the family and traditional society is very protective of them. The honour of the family depends largely on the purity of the daughter before marriage.

Within South Asian culture the elderly have authority and respect. They have an important role within the extended family, for example, counselling the young, arranging marriages, and helping to raise grandchildren. Institutional care and pension systems are essentially non-existent in home countries, and the eldest sons become the guardians of ageing parents.

MARRIAGE

Traditional marriages are arranged. The background and status of the two families are matched, the horoscopes of the couple are often examined, and the marriage is considered to be a union between the families, not just the two individuals. The woman goes to live with her husband's family. Girls are taught from the start that they are temporary members of their families waiting to be given as a gift to someone else. Thus, at marriage, a girl is given to her husband and becomes a member of his family. She is taught that once given in marriage, she may never leave her husband's home. There is a great deal of support from the families as well as social pressure to make a marriage work.

The dowry system, the giving of gifts by the bride's family to the bridegroom, is practised in South Asian culture. Because the man is the earner and will have to support his wife for the rest of her life, the dowry represents her contribution to the marriage. It can be anything from small household items and clothing to appliances, a car, apartment, or gold jewellery. In some cases, the dowry system is abused and in-laws' demands are unreasonable, causing a major crisis for the bride and her family.

South Asian men expect to marry a girl who is a virgin and who has not been out with other men. Girls are consequently well-protected and not allowed to date. A girl who has dated is considered loose and not a suitable marriage partner.

Girls are married young, preferably between the ages of nineteen and twenty-three. The belief is that the bride's adaptation to her husband's family's home will be easier if she has not developed her personality to the fullest extent. If she is young she will be more flexible and adaptable. Similarly, if she has not dated other men she will be more likely to accept the husband her parents have chosen for her. In general, a South Asian man does not expect to make any changes or adjustments when he marries because it is his family and life that his wife is entering.

For the most part, marriages among South Asians in Canada continue to be arranged. Many families look for marriage partners, especially brides for their sons, in home countries rather than in Canada. It is felt that young women who have grown up here have had too much freedom to accept an arranged marriage and entry into a new extended family. There is also a belief that because divorces are common in Canada, a marriage has a better chance of survival and stability if the partner has a more traditional background. Although caste is generally said to be unimportant for Hindu South

Asians in Canada, inter-caste marriages are still unusual. This can create conflicts with young adults who have grown up here and who do not respect the caste system.

Traditionally, South Asian widows did not remarry. Now, however, if a woman is still young, that is, under about thirty years of age, her in-laws or parents may arrange another marriage for her. In general, though, remarriage for widows (and female divorcees) is uncommon.

SEPARATION AND DIVORCE

Both separation and divorce are extremely rare in traditional South Asian society. There is a strong cultural pressure on the couple, especially the wife, to stay together. A woman is brought up to believe that she should never leave her husband's home, and most of the responsibility of making or breaking a home is placed on the woman. The families of both husband and wife will become deeply involved if there are marital problems, as separation and divorce stigmatize the whole family. In traditional society, for example, the unmarried brothers and sisters of a woman who had left her husband and returned home would find it difficult to arrange marriages with suitable families. Parents of the couple and sometimes a respected religious leader will try to resolve problems and decide who is at fault, and every attempt is made to reconcile the couple.

The issue of dowry can sometimes cause the breakup of a marriage in that the husband and his family may feel cheated. For example, a woman who sponsors her husband's immigration to Canada, may feel that no further dowry is necessary. However, his parents, when they immigrate to join them later, may begin to resent her family for not giving a bigger dowry. Or, a girl who comes from India to marry a man here may not bring household goods with her as she has to travel so far, and this may be held against her by her husband's family.

In Canada, the cultural constraints on a couple to stay together at all costs, combined with the stresses of living in an unfamiliar culture, can sometimes result in violence. If a woman were abused by her husband in her home country, her family would step in to protect and support her. If she left her husband, his parents might guarantee her safety and take responsibility for his conduct after her return to him. In Canada, a woman may expect a social worker or counsellor to assume the role of ensuring her safety in the home. Sometimes in Canada people from the same town or village as a woman with marital problems, may mediate for her, in the absence of her parents and relatives. They take responsibility for her and decide what is in her best interests. Friends usually become involved in cases where a woman has no relatives. In such instances, a woman becomes indebted to them and is obligated to follow their advice.

A South Asian woman who has separated from her husband is unlikely to initiate divorce proceedings because she is identified as being the one who left the home or the relationship. It is more acceptable for a man to leave his wife and children, and to initiate a divorce. If a woman leaves her children with her husband, she is considered a bad mother, except in the case of a Muslim family, where custody of the children is assumed by the husband's family. Sometimes even after divorce, a couple will continue in many ways as if still married. A man may occasionally stay with his ex-wife and children, and the community continues to address them as husband and wife.

CHILD-REARING

In South Asian culture, there is a preference for male children who have important ritual functions and are also responsible for care of the parents in their old age. It is important to see that daughters are well-settled so that they will not cause concern in the future. Boys, then, are favoured and receive more attention than girls; the eldest male is the most privileged. The eldest female sibling is given a great deal of responsibility and this can be very demanding.

Independence is not encouraged, especially in girls, and young children may not have much experience of being away from parents or relatives. Pre-school children may use baby talk. In general, there are no fixed schedules for young children; a child goes to bed when he is tired, eats when he is hungry, and so on. As boys and girls grow older, they are discouraged from playing together.

Spanking is not uncommon as a form of discipline and parents may use threats of physical punishment to control behaviour. Children may be given treats to avoid tension and behaviour problems. For example, to avoid a temper tantrum, a child may be given candy. In some cases, to avoid parental punishment, children threaten to call in social workers or other "help lines" to lay complaints of physical abuse. This frightens parents, who may feel that they are losing control over their offspring.

In general, children from South Asian homes are more strictly controlled by their families than are Canadian children. Teenage boys are given more freedom than girls as they will be the earners in the household and must learn to deal with the outside world. In Canada, teenage boys may be expected to take part-time jobs after school to contribute to the family income. On the other hand, girls are very protected and are not allowed to date. In some families, a girl may be expected to come straight home from school and may not have the freedom, for example, to go shopping with friends, to use the local library, or to go to summer camp.

In some cases, parents take on two jobs and work long hours, leaving children relatively unsupervised. Older children may be given the responsibility of baby-sitting younger ones.

Parents want children to be well-educated and a high priority is placed on schooling. However, in home countries, it is the role of the teacher to teach and thus there is little or no parental involvement in schools. Consequently, South Asian parents new to Canada may not be used to participating in school activities or consulting with teachers. For some parents extracurricular activities and social development may be considered unimportant and a waste of their children's time. Parents may expect teachers to take responsibility for disciplining children as is the case in home countries. New immigrants, both students and parents, are likely to find the Canadian school system very different from what they experienced at home. The atmosphere is generally much more lax and liberal. The fact that children receive sex education in Canadian schools may upset some parents, who believe that sexual matters should not be discussed in front of children or adolescents, especially girls. Whereas in South Asian culture children are taught that it is rude and disrespectful to argue with parents or teachers, in Canadian schools children learn that they have a right to voice their opinions and are encouraged to do so. As a result, South Asian children face a conflict between the values of Canadian society and those of their parents.

ROLE CHANGES AND CONFLICTS RESULTING FROM MIGRATION

The process of migration and adjustment to a new culture can impose stresses on the South Asian family structure. For example, traditionally the man is the bread-winner while his wife stays at home. However, because of economic necessity, many South Asian women in Canada must find employment outside the home. This change can be threatening to a traditional husband, who may feel that his wife is becoming too Westernized and, perhaps, having too much contact with other men. He may react by attempting to increase his control over her and she may respond by rebelling. This problem of control and rebelliousness can become so serious that the husband will resort to violence. The experience of employment for women often results in their increased independence and assertiveness which husbands may again find threatening to their traditional dominance. The increased sense of independence may in turn cause women to be less willing to tolerate traditional marital and in-law conduct. Moreover, external employment places an additional strain on women who often must continue to shoulder the sole responsibility for the care of home and family.

A woman who immigrates to Canada in order to marry into a local South Asian family may find herself isolated and without support. She will miss the help of her own family during the period of adjustment to her in-laws' home and will be without their aid in the event of marital problems. Often these women are afraid to gossip and thus do not confide in anyone.

The traditional dominance of the elderly within the family is frequently weakened after moving to Canada. Usually sponsored by a son or daughter, elderly people arrive here in a dependent role, not knowing the language or the culture. With their married children running the home they lose their traditional position of domestic control. This reversal of traditional patterns of dependence and authority can cause conflicts and, a loss of self-esteem and depression in the elderly. Especially in situations where both parents are working, the elderly person may be given the responsibility of housework and baby-sitting. Family members who are preoccupied with becoming established may have little time to devote to ageing parents who lack the linguistic skills and confidence to venture out on their own. The contrast between the social liveliness of the family compound or village and the isolation of the suburban single-family home leaves many elderly South Asians in Canada feeling lonely, saddened, and isolated. In some cases, elderly parents are encouraged to take on outside jobs such as berry-picking or delivering flyers. Their earnings are then added to the family income.

South Asian children and adolescents are often caught between traditional cultural values and practices and those of Canadian society. For example, the experience of the Canadian school system which teaches freedom of thought, individuality, and independent decisionmaking, stands in direct contrast to South Asian extended family values where the family unit's needs are more important than the individual's. Young adults who have grown up in Canada may have difficulty in accepting arranged marriages. South Asian teenage girls who are not allowed to date may be torn between peer pressure at school and traditional parental expectations. These conflicts can lead to rebellion and depression.

Children are sometimes used as interpreters by parents who are not fluent in English. This role can be demanding and stressful for a child who, for example, accompanies his father to the bank to arrange a mortgage. Where he is unable to interpret through lack of understanding, he is likely to feel inadequate and depressed. A pattern of reliance on children for interpretation or for other tasks (such as filling out income tax forms) can lead to role reversal where children lose respect for parents while parents lose authority and control.

Traditionally, conflicts are resolved within the family or community and outsiders are not involved. Where a teenager is misbehaving for example, and the immediate family cannot get him to change his ways, another relative may be called in to help. However, in Canada, children may question the authority of family members who are not part of the nuclear unit: "What has my uncle to do with my business?"

CULTURAL VALUES AND BEHAVIOUR

South Asian names vary with religion and region. Women take their husband's surname at the time of marriage. Hindus generally have three names: a personal name followed by a complimentary name, and then a family name. However, many women have dropped the middle name after coming to Canada. Sikhs typically have three names: a personal name, then a title (Singh for men, Kaur for women), followed by the family name. Examples are, Mohinder Singh Sandhu or Raminder Kaur Gill.

Traditional clothing for women varies from one region to another. Many South Asian women wear a sari, a straight piece of cloth draped around the body like a long dress. Typically, Sikh and Muslim women from northern India and Pakistan wear full trousers beneath a long overblouse, sometimes with a long scarf over the shoulders. In Canada, some women continue to dress traditionally while others, especially those in the work place, adopt Western clothing. Many women, particularly the elderly, prefer slacks to skirts or dresses, to ensure that their legs are covered. Originally, traditional South Asian clothing indicated the wearer's regional background, but today it is current fashion that often dictates style. Traditionally, South Asian women do not cut their hair; Sikh women especially do not cut it for religious reasons. Women who are second or third generation in Canada are more likely to cut their hair and to wear Western style clothing, particularly if they are educated and work in offices or in a profession. Many Sikh men wear turbans and are likely to have beards.

The traditional form of greeting is with the palms of the hands pressed together in front of the chest. Shaking hands, particularly by women, is not common. Customarily, eye contact is considered rude and disrespectful, especially with elders. Physical expressions of affection, such as hugging and kissing, are rare in public, even among family members and close friends. Indeed they are considered extremely inappropriate between members of the opposite sex, including husband and wife. The opinions of relatives and other members of the community are held in high regard and gossip can be used to effect social control.

For people who have come from rural areas, recreation tends to be family- and community-centred. Men go out to meet friends but very few women from rural backgrounds go out alone to socialize, unless it is to meet other women at their homes, or to visit the temple to prepare for weddings or other community celebrations. Gatherings in the home tend to be segregated by sex, with women in one room and men in another. Some wives may insist that their husbands only consume alcohol at social activities away from the home.

It is a not uncommon living arrangement in extended families for children up to the age of twelve to share a bedroom with their parents or with siblings of the opposite sex.

TRADITIONAL BELIEFS ABOUT ILLNESS

All over South Asia many people view illness in quite similar ways, and these derive originally from Ayurvedic medicine, the ancient Indian medical system. Illnesses are the result of imbalance in the body humours, bile, wind, and phlegm, and the purpose of treatment is to re-establish the balance. An imbalance in humours can result from various sources, but dietary imbalance is probably the most common cause of illness. For example, a headache may be explained as the result of eating too many eggs, which are believed to be "heating" foods. Working in the hot sun is also believed to lead to imbalance and illnesses. Immorality and other kinds of excess, be it alcohol, sex, or study, explain other diseases. Finally, possession by a demon or the "evil eye" of a jealous neighbour account for still others, particularly mental illnesses.

A variety of traditional treatments exists to rebalance the

humours. Most commonly, these are herbal decoctions that can be made at home, for example, various teas made by grinding herbs or spices which are boiled with liquids. Often, too, specific foods are used to re-establish bodily balance. Foods in South Asia are classified as "hot," "cold," or "neutral," not in terms of temperature or spiciness but on other grounds. (There is no universally agreed-upon classification; what constitutes cold food varies from one community to another.) Bathing (or its avoidance), massage, and rubbing oil on the body are other ways to rebalance and thus to cure.

Other forms of traditional treatment are directed towards the supernatural causes of illness. In South Asian villages it is often people in stressful circumstances whose troubles are explained supernaturally. For example, the newly married girl who leaves her own village to live with her husband and his parents may find the stress intolerable, particularly if she is overworked and her mother-in-law is unsympathetic. For this and similar illnesses, ritual chanting is performed by an exorcist or a priest who has been especially called to the patient's home. This procedure may end, for example, with the tying of a protective thread around the sick person's wrist, by writing a protective verse to be worn in a metal cylinder on a chain around the neck, or by inscribing religious verses on the patient's hands. A sick person may also make promises of gifts to a temple god if he recovers. Throughout South Asia it is felt that many avenues are available to treat illness. Traditional medicines, vows, rituals, biomedicine may all work, and all may be used for the same illness.

Even though many South Asians, particularly educated urbanites, may not believe in such traditional medicines, many of their habits, remedies, food combinations, and the day-to-day methods of preventing illness are based on these traditional beliefs.

TRADITIONAL TREATMENT IN INDIA

In South Asia traditional medical practitioners are readily available to almost everyone. Particularly in rural villages, the Ayurvedic physician, often a barber who also specializes in bone-setting, or in treating snake-bites, is within walking distance and is usually the first to be consulted. The same applies to other religiously based practitioners and astrologers. An Ayurvedic doctor, often trained as an apprentice, will usually talk with a patient and his family together (Western-style "privacy" is usually not a concern), will sometimes take the patient's pulse or use a biomedical tool like a stethoscope to diagnose the illness, and then will prescribe herbal medicines or recommend bathing or soothing oils. The consultation time is usually short. Since fees or gifts for traditional health services are customary, many rural families try home remedies first. The tendency, particularly in rural villages and among the poor, is to wait until an illness is serious before professional care is sought from outside the village. The reason for this is that money and time are usually in short supply, not because people are fatalistic and believe there is nothing to be done.

Traditional medical services are available in urban areas as well, sometimes in more organized forms such as Ayurvedic hospitals and clinics. Although traditional healers are much more readily available than biomedical doctors, in many parts of South Asia this is not the only reason for choosing to use them. Many South Asians believe that traditional medicine is more natural, slower acting, not as strong, and has fewer side-effects than biomedicine. It is therefore preferred particularly for chronic illnesses where a quick cure is neither important nor expected.

Some South Asians in Canada are likewise hesitant to use biomedicine. Many feel, too, that traditional treatments are more effective than biomedicine for certain diseases, such as rheumatism or asthma. For that reason even urban, well-educated people may prefer traditional medicine for some symptoms.

BIOMEDICAL SYSTEM IN SOUTH ASIA

India has one biomedical physician for 3,640 people, in contrast to Canada's one doctor per 550 people. Other South Asian countries are similar (World Bank 1983). There may sometimes be a biomedical physician in a larger village who serves surrounding villages as well. Some villages may also have untrained "doctors" who give injections and supply Western-type drugs. More commonly, though, biomedical physicians practise in towns and cities. Since health insurance is essentially unavailable in South Asia, everyone must pay for physicians' services and medicines, the latter usually being dispensed in the doctor's office. Thus a visit to a biomedical doctor is very expensive for village families and is avoided unless the disease is serious and the family can afford the fees, medicines, and travel expenses.

Many South Asian villages, however, have trained and untrained midwives who deliver babies at home and provide pre- and postnatal care. Their services may include supervising delivery, giving advice about diet and behaviour, performing suitable rituals, and bathing and caring for mother and baby for some time after birth. Midwives are paid in cash or with gifts of food and clothing.

That hospitals are only used for more serious illnesses is suggested by the statistics; India has only one hospital bed per 1,310 people, in contrast to one bed per 110 persons in Canada. Hospitals are usually located in towns and cities remote from many villages. When a village family does go to hospital, no appointments are made and hospital staff are often very busy. Unless families know someone working at the hospital to whom they can appeal for help (a common way of dealing with such problems), patients and their families must take a number or wait in a queue, sometimes for several hours. When they finally see a physician there is little time for extensive taking of histories or for answering the patient's questions. Instead, the physician usually diagnoses quickly and decides immediately on treatment. It is only the urban, middle-class people who emigrate from South Asia to Canada who will have experienced hospitals and physicians similar to those in Canada.

DISEASE IN SOUTH ASIA

While there is a substantial urban middle-class in South Asia with satisfactory incomes and access to good health care, the large proportion of the South Asian population is poor. Incomes are low and uncertain, houses crowded, water supplies unprotected, sanitation inadequate, and nutrition poor. The generally low standard of living is evident in the fact that a person born in 1981 could expect to live fifty-two years in South Asia, but seventy-five years in Canada. In India, too, infant mortality during the first year of life is very high with 121 deaths for every 1,000 babies. In Canada the equivalent figure is 10 per 1,000.

Infections and parasitic diseases are the most prevalent in South Asia. Consequently, some South Asian immigrants to Canada may have experienced typhoid, dengue fever, cholera, tuberculosis, hepatitis, and amoebic dysentry. Of particular relevance is malaria. Although there have been relatively effective programs to eradicate this scourge, the incidence of malaria in India has increased recently, from a low of 100,000 cases and no deaths in 1965 to a high of six million cases in 1976. The area of greatest resurgence is Gujarat, where some Canadian immigrants originate. Moreover, malaria is particularly common in many cities. The incidence of heart disease, cancer, stroke, and diabetes, is relatively low, and is to be expected in a country whose inhabitants have a relatively low life expectancy.

Documented diseases among South Asian immigrants in the Western world are malaria, tuberculosis (including types other than pulmonary), several types of intestinal parasite, filarisis, vitamin A deficiency, and rickets.

SEEKING HEALTH CARE IN SOUTH ASIA AND CANADA

In cases of sickness in South Asian villages, it is not simply the victim who decides on a suitable course of action. Instead, the whole family may be consulted (and sometimes neighbours) and the final decision about the need to spend money on a visit to a doctor may rest with the head of the household. For example, when a child falls sick, the mother will often consult her mother-in-law about appropriate home remedies. The mother-in-law or household head will also decide if the child should be taken to a doctor or hospital. Many factors influence the decision, including cost and time but also the identity of the sick person. A wage-earner may be much more promptly treated than others, and a first-born son more quickly than a daughter.

Among South Asian villagers who have emigrated to Canada, the extended family often remains strong so that the old ways of making health decisions persist, particularly in the initial phase. Elderly women often recommend home treatments and the elderly members and the male household head are consulted about the need to see a doctor.

Especially in their early days in Canada, village families do not decide to use physicians on a regular basis but only for acute illnesses. In choosing a family physician, language familiarity is often important, but so are proximity and convenience for the mother.

TRADITIONAL MEDICINE IN CANADA

When South Asian villagers first come to Canada, resort to traditional medicines often continues, even where the family has health insurance and easy access to biomedicine. Home remedies such as massage, bathing, and herbal medicines (either made at home or purchased from an Indian shop) may be used first, while a physician is sought out only for serious illnesses. Advertisements in some local South Asian newspapers reveal that traditional astrologers and palm readers also operate in Canada. Sometimes traditional treatments are used concomitantly with biomedicines or are preferred because

Western-style medicines are believed to have unpleasant side effects and to be too strong.

While greater variation exists among longer-term South Asian inhabitants of Canada, there are still many who adhere to traditional tonics and ointments. And many more eat specific combinations of foods to prevent or treat illness, sometimes without knowing the theory behind the practice. Often South Asians who are well educated and think of themselves as modern or Westernized are reluctant to discuss their use of traditional treatments.

RELATIONSHIP BETWEEN DOCTOR AND PATIENT

In South Asia, patients and families often put great trust in both traditional and modern physicians. The patient may expect the doctor to have all the answers and make all the decisions. As a result the patient takes a passive role, answering but not asking questions, and waits for the physician to impart his diagnosis and recommendations. Medical advice is often accepted without question. Further, social distance between South Asian doctors and most patients is very great so that the relationship is formal. Patients typically use deferential forms of address.

It is also expected that the doctor will go beyond asking questions. He will examine the patient by taking his pulse and temperature or looking down his throat. Moreover, the patient expects palpable treatment in the form of medicine, injections, pills, or tonics. Failing this, the patient will be dissatisfied with the treatment and will lack confidence in the doctor.

These expectations can often create dissatisfaction among South Asian patients in Canada when they consult physicians trained in the West. A doctor who says, "I do not know what is wrong. We need to do more tests," or "Come back the next time that symptom recurs so that we can investigate," may be perceived as incompetent. Also, a doctor who asks the patient, "What would you like me to do about it?" may be regarded in the same light as the physician who says, "It is just a cold. There is no need for medicine." Doctors who behave and dress informally may also disappoint South Asian expectations. An active and commanding doctor who takes charge and gives medical prescriptions may be preferred by many South Asians.

South Asian women tend to be hesitant and shy about being examined and treated by male physicians and both they and their husbands believe that women should have a female doctor. In South Asia, however, there is often no choice and in Canada convenience of access is often a more important criterion than the doctor's sex except in the case of obstetricians, who should preferably be women.

HOSPITALIZATION

Visiting

For many rural South Asians hospitalization occurs only when illness is severe and often involves travelling to relatively distant towns. Family members may stay with the patient in hospital or visit daily to help with nursing tasks. Also, many families will bring food which they believe to be better than hospital fare. Relatives, friends, and neighbours, including children, make great efforts to express their concern for the patient and the family by making hospital visits.

These practices continue in Canada. Family, friends, and neighbours want to visit a hospitalized person and the patient welcomes their attention. The patient will more likely feel happy than tired after a visit by a crowd of people, and may be dismayed if certain people do not appear. Visiting hours often take on the atmosphere of a family reunion with much food, talking, laughing, and eating. It is not enough to drop by briefly. Instead, visitors—both friends and family—are expected to sit and spend time with the patient.

Understandably, South Asian family members are sometimes disturbed when forbidden to visit the patient, for example, in intensive care units. In this case, it is not uncommon for family and friends to gather outside in a corridor, simply in order to be together near the patient. For many South Asians, hospital visits are a very important way to provide support for both the sick person and his family. Hospital visits are believed to be right and proper by most South Asians, both in South Asia and in Canada.

Large numbers of visitors, lengthy visits, and gifts of food are often in breach of the culture-bound rules of many Canadian hospitals. If limiting the number of visitors is desired, the hospital staff can most easily approach the patient's husband, father, or a male elder to explain the situation and to seek the co-operation of the others.

Hospital Food

Canadian hospital food can present problems for South Asians, particularly those who strictly observe religious dietary restrictions. For example, a vegetarian may not accept a vegetarian meal if it was prepared in a kitchen where meat was also cooked, or if the meat has simply been removed from the plate.

Hospital food is too bland for most South Asians. In addition, since many South Asians hold that food and particular illnesses are causally interrelated, they may be reluctant to eat some items, but may readily suggest suitable substitutes.

Hospital Clothing

Some South Asian patients in Canada hesitate to wear clothing that others have worn before them, even where it has been washed and sterilized. They prefer their own clothing where possible. South Asian women may prefer not to use hospital clothing for new babies since they may be particularly superstitious about the harmful effects of used clothing.

Hospital Treatments and Surgery

Although many South Asians accept the doctor's authority to prescribe treatment, surgery is sometimes felt to be threatening. Only after detailed explanations about the surgical procedure and its necessity, will the family agree. In some cases where surgery is refused, the decision is made not by the individual patient but by the whole family, and the patient will be taken home. In other instances the family may agree but will suggest an auspicious day for surgery on the basis of an astrologer's predictions.

There is no religious or other belief that prevents blood transfusions or organ transplants.

However, some religious practices exist that hospital staff should know about when treating South Asian patients. High-caste Hindu men participate in a religious ceremony at adolescence in which a sacred thread (or string) is tied around the body; it goes over one shoulder around the chest and is tied at waist-level. Because of its religious significance, this thread should not be cut or removed without the permission of the patient or his family. Strictly observant Sikh men do not cut their hair. If it must be cut it is important to explain the need fully both to the patient and the family. The Sikh man's bracelet and kirpan must also not be removed. Muslims sometimes wear thirty-three beads around their necks or wrists, and these represent the ninety-nine names of God. They should not be removed unless absolutely necessary.

Most South Asians prefer that catheterization or enemas be performed by a staff member of the same sex as the patient.

Some Indian bathing and toilet practices can be troublesome since many hospitals lack suitable equipment and procedures.

USE OF MEDICINES

The concern that biomedicines may be too strong or upset the body's balance leads many South Asian patients to avoid their use or stop taking them prematurely. This is true of all types of medicines, but especially long-term psychiatric medicines. Once the person begins to feel better he or she stops taking them, since "If you're taking medicine you must still be sick."

MENTAL ILLNESS

In South Asia, mental illness is sometimes believed to have supernatural causes, particularly spells or curses cast by jealous relatives or acquaintances. These problems are resolved by visiting temples or shrines. Astrologers may also be consulted for a prognosis of the problem. Symptoms of mental illness are usually presented to a physician in somatic form, for example, as headaches, stomachaches, and burning bodily sensations, rather than as anxiety or depression. Such somatic complaints are more acceptable in part because mental illness is stigmatized, and is generally hidden to safeguard the children's marriage arrangements.

Many of these beliefs and practices persist in the South Asian community in Canada. Severely ill family members are not ignored or rejected, but may be kept hidden and thus may remain untreated for long periods of time, only to arrive at hospital emergency rooms by ambulance or police car after uncontrollable outbreaks or suicide attempts. Less severe psychiatric symptoms like depression or neurosis are thought of as somatic complaints and presented to a doctor with a request for medicine. In some instances South Asian families will seek explanations from palm readers, astrologers, and other healers who practice in Canada. Such is the case of the parents who decided that their daughter-in-law had cast a chanting spell on their son, because he listened only to her. Where the problems are serious and the family has the money, they may return to their home country for rituals and charms.

When a South Asian family moves to the West there are a number of common problems, mostly related to leaving home and living in a new culture, that seem to precipitate psychiatric symptoms. Because education is felt to be important to upward mobility in

Canada, failing a school examination may be devastating for a young person. Also, adolescents and young adults often face an insoluble dilemma in trying to balance traditional parental expectations against more liberal peer group pressures. Thus the young South Asian girl may have two identities, one for home and one for school. The resulting stress and guilt may lead to depression which, if severe, may end in suicide attempts using, for example, household poisons. Disturbed family relationships may also precipitate psychiatric illness. Often the arrival of a mother-in-law from Asia or conflict between husband and wife over financial and other obligations to their respective families creates stress and symptoms.

While most South Asians treat these problems as somatic and prefer medicines, some patients in Canada do resort to psychiatric help. Western "talk" therapy is not usually compatible with South Asian beliefs or expectations, especially initially. The preference is for clear and authoritative advice about what the patient should do and how the family should help. The usual open ended psychiatric interviewing method and its assumption that the patient must be helped to find his or her own solutions does not accord with South Asian expectations that the physician is in command. Attempts to elicit the family circumstances of the South Asian patient are not usually welcomed since family harmony is usually more highly prized than individual well-being. The therapeutic value often attached to independence from the family in the West is not usually acceptable to Indian psychiatric patients.

Many South Asian families are more willing and able to use the advice and help of community agencies and schools than that of psychiatrists or the mental health system, especially when the sick person is an adolescent. Help that is provided in an informal and egalitarian way is generally more effective.

PREGNANCY

In South Asia, pregnancy is considered a normal, healthy state. Consequently many women do not see the need to consult a doctor unless there is a problem. This is particularly true of women in rural areas, who usually plan on home deliveries. Help and advice is provided by the pregnant woman's mother or mother-in-law as well as by a midwife who usually visits periodically.

Life continues as usual throughout pregnancy. Couples continue sexual relations. Women who ordinarily work in the fields continue to do so, although they may avoid lifting heavy objects. In general the woman's diet remains the same although she will avoid hot foods such as meat, eggs, and nuts, especially during the first trimester as they are believed to cause miscarriage or premature delivery. Thus emphasis is on cooling foods such as some fruit, coconut, yogurt, butter and milk, which may be eaten in increased quantity, particularly butter and milk.

There is a strong preference for male children among South Asian families, particularly for the first child. Consequently there has in India been a recent increase in requests for amniocentesis by urban Indian women to determine the sex of the unborn child. Requests for abortion sometimes follow if the child is female.

In Canada, some South Asian women believe regular check-ups during pregnancy to be unimportant. Indeed, they may be avoided, or cause anxiety because visits to a doctor are associated with problems or abnormalities. Also, a young woman in Canada may be deterred from obtaining prenatal care by traditionalist relatives, in-laws, or mothers, who may discourage "new" practices, saying "I have the experience of giving birth to ten or twelve children and can advise my daughter. Is there anything new about childbirth here?"

While many South Asian women are encouraged to attend prenatal classes by physicians and public health nurses, most prefer not to go for a variety of reasons. Language is often a problem, and many of the teachings offend the woman's idea of propriety. Sex is discussed openly with strangers and movies of childbirth are shown, both of which make many South Asian women uncomfortable. Also, they are embarassed about doing exercises in front of other people. Their husbands tend to feel even more embarassed and uncomfortable in these classes and thus usually refuse to attend.

Some South Asian women who are recent immigrants may experience considerable stress during pregnancy, especially when they have married a man who is a relative stranger. In addition to the typical adjustments to a new language, culture, in-law family, and husband, she may become pregnant immediately and suffer from morning sickness. Unable to confide in her husband or mother-in-law and with no family of her own, she may keep things to herself, lose weight, and receive little sympathy or help. Both emotional and physical stress result.

An unmarried girl who becomes pregnant is often rejected by her family since virginity at marriage is highly valued, and lack of it greatly complicates marriage arrangements. In Canada, where financial aid is available to single mothers, it is possible for the rejected South Asian girl to live independently. Even so, the loss of family and cultural support is often intolerable.

CHILDBIRTH

In South Asia the woman traditionally returned to her own parents'
home for delivery of her first child, and sometimes for subsequent
births. Although this is changing, most births still occur at home,
supervised by midwives in the presence of the woman's mother,
mother-in-law, or married sister. Childbirth is considered to be a
woman's business and husbands participate only in so far as they
stay near the house in case of emergency. During labour the midwife
often encourages the woman to be active, to walk around, and sometimes gives the woman herbal medicines to facilitate the process.
Delivery is often in a squatting or sitting position. The baby remains
with the mother after birth.

In Canada, where hospital deliveries are the norm, many practices
will be unfamiliar to a woman who has previously had children in
South Asia. However, she will of course have talked to her friends
and have some idea about what will happen. Her husband usually
accompanies her to the hospital but prefers to stay out of the delivery room. The woman's preference is usually for a natural delivery
so that she will not generally request an anaesthetic. Such decisions
she would leave to the physician. Forceps and Caesarian section are
usually accepted if clearly explained by the doctor. Those South
Asian women lacking facility in English experience additional stress
during delivery. In these cases the presence of an English-speaking
married female relative or friend is often reassuring.

Asian babies born in the West are, on the average, lower in weight
than white Caucasian babies (2.96 kg versus 3.29 kg), but this difference is not usually the result of maternal malnutrition during pregnancy (Mason et al. 1982).

When a Muslim child is born, religious practice requires that a
family member recite a prayer in the baby's ear as soon as possible.
A male Muslim baby must be circumcised. For other religious
groups circumcision is a matter of personal preference.

South Asian women, accustomed to keeping the baby with them,
may feel concerned at the Canadian practice of placing the baby in a
nursery in certain instances.

The sex of the new-born child is of paramount importance to
many Indian women and their husbands and relatives. For a South
Asian woman the birth of a daughter may occasion crisis and fear of
blame. Emotional outbreaks sometimes occur and in extreme instances neither the woman's husband nor family members will visit the
hospital if the baby is a girl.

After childbirth, particularly if the baby is a boy, visitors will come in large numbers to celebrate the event, bringing sweets for all.

POSTPARTUM PERIOD

The traditional practice in South Asia is for the mother and new baby to remain secluded in the home for a week to forty days, depending on region and caste. The belief is that the woman is at her weakest in this period and is most susceptible to chills, backaches, and the like, and requires rest. Failure by the mother to comply is believed to expose her to arthritis and other illnesses later on. Such periods of seclusion after childbirth are common among Indian women in Canada as well.

Since the new mother is expected to be with the baby to the exclusion of all else, members of her extended family may help or a relative may come to stay for a month or so.

During the postpartum period South Asian women are advised to eat hot foods and to avoid cold ones. It is believed that heating foods strengthen the body, regulate the system, and encourage bleeding and discharge so that a flat stomach results. Cold foods cause weight gain. One snack commonly eaten by Punjabi women during this period is panjiri, a whole wheat flour fried in butter with sugar, almonds, pistachios, raisins, and several kinds of seeds. All of these are heating ingredients. It is important to keep warm, avoid fans, and to keep well covered even in hot weather. Bathing is acceptable, but the water must be warm. Vigorous massages with oil are also used.

During the forty-day period visitors are welcome and may bring gifts or cash. The new parents may also have a party to celebrate the birth. However, certain people do not visit since they bring bad luck to the baby: widows, women who have lost children, and people in mourning. To avoid harm to the child, visitors are careful not to compliment or admire the baby to excess, lest parents worry about the effects of the evil eye.

A woman is considered unclean in this postpartum period and the couple abstains from sexual relations. At the conclusion of this seclusion she takes a special bath, and rituals are performed to mark the return to a clean state.

BREAST-FEEDING

In South Asia, in both rural and urban areas, breast-feeding is preferred, although the baby may be bottle-fed where the middle-class mother has to return to her job. Generally, though, women breast-feed for at least six months and sometimes up to two or three years. In Canada, some South Asian women prefer to bottle-feed, partly because they believe it to be "modern." Some may bottle-feed simply to allow their mother-in-law the pleasure of feeding the new baby. Husbands, too, may influence the choice between breast-feeding or bottle-feeding. Some children are given a bottle up to ages three or four.

FAMILY PLANNING

In South Asia, particularly in rural areas, where children are needed to help with farm work, families are large; eight to ten children in a family is not unusual. Children are believed to be God's gift and are welcomed. While couples have always known ways of preventing birth, abstinence and withdrawal being the most common, the modern methods of birth control are still not commonly used, especially by village people.

Families that come to Canada, or are started here, tend to be smaller than the norm because women have less help at home, often have jobs, and because the cost of raising children is greater. Modern methods of controlling births are more acceptable and are used, but more often after the desired number of children has been born rather than to space births. The first child, usually born within the first year of marriage, is important because it demonstrates the wife's fertility to the husband and his family. Several closely spaced pregnancies follow, but marital stress can occur where only daughters are born. Often it is the husband who makes decisions about family size. The favourite methods of contraception are the IUD and contraceptive pill; diaphragms and condoms are seldom used. Women tend to believe that breast-feeding automatically protects against conception.

South Asian women are not usually comfortable about discussing family planning or sexuality with a nurse or doctor, especially if their husbands or mothers are present. They usually talk more easily in private.

Abortion is thought of as killing the child and is thus not generally accepted by South Asians either overseas or in Canada. However, illegal abortion is practised in South Asia and may be resorted to in desperate situations such as when an unmarried girl becomes pregnant. Abortion in Canada is somewhat more acceptable to South Asian couples, particularly if the woman is ill, if they cannot afford another child, or where pregnancies are very closely spaced. However, the decision is not just the woman's and her physician's, but requires her husband's approval and perhaps his family's.

DISABILITY AND REHABILITATION

A South Asian family may find difficulty in accepting a handicapped child or in helping it in the ways that the Western health system expects. As with mental illness, some disabilities may be hidden because they reflect on the whole family, and some parents account for the situation in terms of karma. Some handicaps may be explained in either religious or supernatural terms and the disabled person is taken to shrines and temples for ritual prayers. Thus, disability may be understood in fatalistic terms, rather than being seen as a medical problem for which helpful treatment may exist.

A handicap in a daughter is seen as a special problem by her parents because she may be prevented from marrying, and will remain a lifelong burden on them.

Many South Asian families are likely to accept and foster the dependence of handicapped members, pitying them and helping them rather than encouraging them to greater independence, particularly if initial rehabilitation efforts produce little improvement. Exercises, independent social activities, and other rehabilitative activities advocated by the medical services may be disregarded simply because the South Asian family does not see independence as important or relevant.

Dental Health

In rural areas in South Asia dentists are rarely used. Instead, a villager may use home remedies (for example, a whole clove) for a toothache, pull the tooth himself, or go to a traditional practitioner. Customarily, village people chew on a twig from the neem tree to clean their teeth daily. When South Asians come to Canada most use toothbrushes but sometimes only irregularly and a dentist may be consulted for acute pain. But regular visits to a dentist are not common, mainly because many families cannot afford to pay for services that are not covered by medical insurance.

BATHING AND ELIMINATION

There is a general belief in South Asia that bathing in still water (as in a bathtub) is unclean and thus South Asians generally use running water, such as a stream, a shower, or by pouring buckets of clean water over their bodies. The same preference for showers is found in Canada, and is one that is sometimes not met in Canadian hospitals. South Asian patients would probably prefer a pitcher of water or a private area by a sink to the usual bath.

Some South Asian people do not use toilet paper but wash their bodies with clean water, using the left hand only (the right hand is traditionally used for eating). In South Asia and in South Asian homes in Canada, a water tap or a bucket of clean water is usually available next to the toilet along with a pint-sized plastic pitcher or dipping bowl. In Canadian hospitals, many Indian patients would prefer to have a container of water and a bowl or pitcher provided in the toilet area or with the bedpan.

FOOD AND NUTRITION

Food has very important implications for religion and health in South Asia. Hot and cold foods, and the balance between them, can cause or cure illnesses. Certain foods are prohibited by the main religions, food preparation may be important, and there are times and situations when fasting is required.

Hindu Food Practices

Strict Hindus practice the doctrine of non-violence against living things and thus abstain from meat or fish. The more orthodox, especially women, do not even eat eggs. Because the cow is sacred, Hindus do not eat beef, veal, beef extract, or any other form of beef. Dairy products are, however, considered pure although strict vegetarians do not eat Western cheese because it is made with animal rennet. Pork is forbidden because it is considered unclean. Strict vegetarians will be unhappy if served vegetarian items from the same plate or with the same utensils that have been used for meat. Alcohol is not prohibited but should be used in moderation only.

The Hindu caste system dictates that members of one caste cannot sit down to eat with members of another nor eat food prepared or served by a lower caste member.

Fasting is used as a self-sacrifice to earn religious merit, to ward off evil, and to absolve sins. For example, a pregnant woman who has had two or three daughters might vow to fast for a certain number of days (for example, sixteen Mondays) if her next child is a son. Fasting may take many forms depending on individual interpretation, from total abstinence (no food or water for twenty-four hours) to one meal a day, or to eating only foods considered to be pure (for example, fruit, yogurt, nuts, or potatoes). Once a year many Hindu women fast for their husbands' long life, eating a meal before 5:30 A.M. and then not again until they see the moon that night. Some fast in this way each month or week.

Very few Hindus would insist on fasting when ill or in hospital, and even they would probably agree to take hot milk, fruit, tea, and salad without salt.

Hindus living in Canada vary a great deal in terms of their adherence to these religious prescriptions.

Muslim Food Practices

Muslims follow dietary laws laid down in the Koran which forbid the eating of pork in any form or eating the blood of any animal. Special methods of slaughtering are used to produce meat that is halal. In Canada, such meat is purchased from a Muslim butcher. Foods containing non-halal meat products are forbidden as are other food cooked in places where pork has been cooked. Only fish with fins or scales are allowed; shellfish are not permissable. Alcohol is also forbidden.

Each year all post-adolescent Muslims observe the month-long fast of Ramadan when no food or beverage is consumed from sunrise to sunset. Young children, ill or journeying people, and women who are menstruating, pregnant, or breast-feeding are exempted but are expected to make a compensatory fast at another time.

Just as with the Hindus, Muslims in Canada differ in their observance of religious rules.

Sikh Food Practices

Although there are no significant dietary restrictions on the Sikh religion, many Sikhs are vegetarians. Traditionally beef and pork are not eaten and smoking and alcohol consumption are discouraged. Some Sikhs also fast.

All of the above dietary restrictions and practices are of importance to many South Asians in Canada. They may refuse food because they do not know whether the food has been made with the acceptable ingredients. In a hospital, South Asians would find it helpful to be told whether dishes served to them contain beef, pork, shellfish, and so on.

Diet and Eating Practices

Despite great regional variation, the commonest staple in South Asia is some sort of cereal, usually rice or unleavened bread made of wheat flour. In the Punjab, from which many Canadian Asians come, many people are vegetarians who eat whole wheat roti, ghee (clarified butter), milk, buttermilk, brown sugar, lentils, seasonal vegetables, and fruit. Normally, in villages, there is an early morning cup of tea followed by a large mid-morning meal and another meal at the end of the day. Urban South Asians may have early tea, a larger breakfast at 9:00 A.M., lunch at 1:00 P.M., tea with sweets or other snacks at 5:00 or 6:00 P.M. and a light supper at 9:00 P.M.. Traditionally South Asians in both rural and urban areas eat with the fingers of the right hand and water is provided to wash the hands before and after the meal.

Babies are not generally given special foods. Instead, solid foods such as soft rice, cream of wheat, mashed bananas, or potatoes will be given some time after the second month, followed by bread, rice, meat, or lentils cooked with some salt but no spices in the ninth or tenth month. By fifteen months, the baby is eating adult foods, including eggs, chapatis, lentils, and rice.

After coming to Canada, it is relatively easy for South Asian families to continue eating familiar foods since ingredients are readily available, at least in the larger cities. However, some junk foods are tempting, both because they are "modern" and because they are convenient for families where many people work on different schedules. The result is sometimes poorer levels of nutrition than previously enjoyed by the family in Asia. Some South Asian mothers also are confused about the relative food merits of various forms of milk (sweetened condensed milk, evaporated milk, yogurt, and so on), to the detriment of their infant's nutrition. Mealtimes change in Canada as well and the South Asian housewife may find herself cooking individual meals for each family member as he or she comes home from work. Most South Asians in Canada are relatively comfortable eating with cutlery in public even though they may not do so at home.

FOOD AND THE PREVENTION OF ILLNESS

Diseases are often held to result from an imbalance between hot and cold within the body. They thus can be prevented or treated by using hot or cold foods to achieve balance. Whether a food is hot or cold is unrelated to temperature or spiciness, and the classification varies from region to region.

Diseases thought of as cold, for example, arthritis, rheumatism, respiratory infections, upset stomach and other gastrointestinal problems, and circulatory problems, are suitably treated with hot foods such as ginger and garlic. Cold foods are also avoided in cases of fever. Instead, hot milk is offered. Following surgery, which is a cold state, cold foods are avoided because they may produce swelling in the affected area. On the other hand, hot foods accelerate healing. If these considerations are neglected, it is believed that the patient may develop pain in the muscles or bones in old age. Colds or other respiratory problems are also believed to be cold diseases and thus the common Western home remedy, fruit juice, is not suitable. In fact it is believed that juices and cold milk will aggravate the condition. For hot states, for example during pregnancy, cold foods are recommended, such as yogurt, milk, and fruit.

It is important for ill people to be given easily digested, soft food such as cream of wheat, lentils without spices, khichari (lentils and rice), and soup made of whole wheat flour and milk. These are the foods a South Asian family might bring a patient in hospital.

Beliefs about hot and cold foods are very strongly embedded in South Asian culture. Even South Asians who have lived in Canada for many years often follow these eating guidelines and modify their diets during illness and childbearing accordingly, by taking care to eat the appropriate combination of foods each day.

USE OF ALCOHOL

In South Asia there are religious restrictions on alcohol consumption and many village people are too poor to afford it, although homemade liquor is produced in many villages. Consequently, some South Asian men may drink but it is unusual for women to do so. When families come to Canada and achieve relative prosperity, alcohol, which is readily available, can become a problem for some men (but not women), particularly where the man is feeling the stress of adapting to a new culture.

Excessive drinking among South Asian men in Canada has given rise to family conflict, misuse of family money and, in some cases, extramarital affairs with non-Asian women. This is not usually defined as a problem requiring outside help until it reaches a crisis. In that case religious or community services are more often acceptable and helpful than is medical treatment.

CARE OF THE ELDERLY

When South Asian parents grow old they expect to be cared for by children, particularly sons, and the sons recognize this obligation. Care is relatively easy in Asia where large families can share the day-to-day burdens. Residence in Canada does not change the expectation, but it often alters the practicability. If husband and wife must both work and there are no other relatives to share the responsibility for care, then the family may agree to place an old person in a nursing home. This will be done only as a last resort, after all other possibilities have been considered.

DEATH AND DYING

Religious and other cultural beliefs support the South Asian's acceptance of death as part of life. For Hindus, there will be another life after death and death is openly discussed by all, including children. Associated with acceptance of death is the idea of fatalism, that death will come when it is time for the person to die. This time may either be preordained by God (among Muslims) or determined by one's karma (among Hindus and Sikhs). Death is not hidden.

While there are specific rituals and practices in each religious community, all South Asians hold some beliefs in common. Death at home is preferred, because the dying person's family can care for him or her and because the appropriate actions can be taken both before and after death. A peaceful death at home, surrounded by family, is strongly preferred to death in hospital, especially as the family may perceive that the dying person is being unnecessarily "tortured" by medical procedures.

In South Asia it is generally not the practice for a physician to inform the patient that he or she will soon die. In Canada this practice is quite common and is seen as threatening to both the South Asian patient and his or her family. Instead, the family might wish to be informed and be allowed to discuss the impending death with a physician. It is unlikely that they would pass on the information to the patient, preferring not to upset him or her. In some cases, of course, the elderly South Asian person may recognize that death is imminent and may talk about it openly and comfortably with relatives.

When death occurs, it is expected that surviving families and friends will express their grief openly, by moaning, crying, and so on. It is rare that a death is taken serenely; a person who does so may become the subject of criticism or gossip.

Hindu Death Rituals and Practices

Before death, relatives of the dying person may bring clothing and money for him to touch before distributing them to the needy. As well, they may sit by the dying person and read from a holy book or chant prayers. Both rituals are believed to be helpful in the person's next life. The dying person may want to look at a picture of a god so that the god will be at the forefront of his or her mind at the time of death.

The eldest surviving son plays an important part in the rituals after death. He, along with other relatives, washes the body and dresses it in new clothing. In the case of a married woman red clothing and jewellery, signifying her married state, are used. When a person dies in a Canadian hospital, the family prefers to wash and dress the body before it is removed from the hospital.

In South Asia and Canada bodies are cremated, usually on the same day as the death, and ashes are kept until they can be thrown on to the surface of the sacred river, the Ganges. In Canada, however, the family may also throw the ashes into a local river or the sea. Traditionally, cremation ceremonies are attended only by men.

A mourning period of forty days follows. For the first eighteen days friends and relatives visit and care for the dead person's family, to help them bear their grief. On the eighteenth day the family provides food for Brahmins and the poor so that the soul of the dead person will rest in peace. Often a further remembrance ceremony occurs one year after the death.

Hindus are reluctant to agree to a post mortem on the body.

Muslim Death Rituals and Practices

As a person nears death, Muslims give important support and encouragement by repeating the words of the *Koran* to the person. At death, grief is shown by way of crying and lamenting.

Once death has occurred, the body is ritually washed before being buried with the face pointing towards Mecca. If death occurs in hospital, it is preferred that staff not wash the body but that they turn the head towards the right shoulder before wrapping the body in a plain sheet. During these procedures family members may wish to read passages of scripture or to make lamentation.

Religious rules stipulate that the body should be buried as soon as possible after death and that it be complete and whole. For these reasons, Muslims will agree to a post mortem only if it is legally necessary, and will request that the organs be returned to the body for burial.

Sikh Death Rituals and Practices

When a Sikh dies, members of his or her family prefer to wash the body and prepare it for cremation. The body is viewed at the hospital if that is where death occurred. Sikh men and women go to the crematorium where the eldest son usually lights the funeral pyre. Open display of emotions is acceptable and even expected. After the cremation there is a memorial service at the Sikh temple, at which time prayers are said for the soul of the person. Often another ceremony is held on the yearly anniversary of the death. Like other South Asians, Sikhs do not readily agree to post mortems nor do they agree to donate organs.

USE OF HEALTH AND SOCIAL SERVICES

In South Asia, and in the many countries from which people of South Asian culture have emigrated, health services are privately run and must be sought out by the people who choose to use them. Government-sponsored social services, such as exist in Canada, are non-existent. Instead, families are expected to help their relatives who are in need of money, household help, and other special care. There is little experience with social service agencies and sometimes distrust of all government servants.

Thus, when South Asian families come to Canada, many find the activities of public health nurses and social workers, for example, unfamiliar and often threatening. In particular, home visits by such people are not always acceptable and South Asian families are likely to use social service agencies only as a last resort, after seeking help from family, friends, the temple, or a physician. Accepting financial help from social agencies is frowned upon and thus only reluctantly accepted.

South Asian communities in Canada have sometimes organized their own culturally acceptable services. In Vancouver, for example, both Sikh and Hindu temples offer a variety of social and community activities, including libraries, meeting rooms, English classes, Indian language classes for children, kitchens and halls for ceremonies and gatherings. OASIS, the Orientation and Adjustment Services for Immigrants Society, provides counselling, information, interpretation, and education for South Asians experiencing family or stress problems. Similar agencies are found in other Canadian cities, and their services may be the most readily acceptable to the Canadian South Asian.

FURTHER READING

Ananth, J. "Treatment of Immigrant Indian Patients," *Canadian Journal of Psychiatry*, Vol. 29 (Oct. 1984): 490–3

Buchignani, Norman and Doreen M. Indra. *Continuous Journey: A Social History of South Asians in Canada*. Toronto: McClelland & Stewart 1985

Jain, S. *East Indians in Canada*. The Hague: Klop Press 1971

Kanungo, Rabindra N., ed. *South Asians in the Canadian Mosaic*. Montreal: Kala Bharati Foundation 1984

Mason, E.S. et al. "Early Post-Natal Weight Gain: Comparison between Asian and White Caucasian Infants," *Early Human Development*, Vol. 6 (1982): 253–5

World Bank: *World Tables*, 3rd ed., Vol. 2, *Social Data* (1983)

CONTRIBUTORS

Parin Dossa (University of Calgary)
Soma Ganesan (Physician, Vancouver General Hospital)
Kuldip Gill (UBC)
Guninder Mumick (Vancouver Health Department)
Kanwal Inder Singh Neel (Richmond)
Joseph Richardson (Ganges, BC)
Rev. Vasant Saklikar (New Westminster)
Dave Sangha (Ministry of Social Services and Housing, Vancouver)
Judita Scott (G.F. Strong Rehabilitation Centre, Vancouver)
Roop Seebaran (UBC)
Merry Wood (UBC)

CHAPTER EIGHT

The Vietnamese

Dai-Kha Dinh, Soma Ganesan, and Nancy Waxler-Morrison

GEOGRAPHY

Vietnam is a small country about one-third the size of British Columbia which has a long eastern boundary along the Pacific Ocean and common borders with China in the north, Laos in the northwest, and Kampuchea (Cambodia) in the southwest. Long and narrow, and shaped like the letter "S," the country is divided into three regions. Northern Vietnam is mainly mountainous with a small delta of the Red River; Central Vietnam is mainly plateau; and South Vietnam is a large alluvial plain along the Mekong River. The climate is tropical and the wet season lasts from May until November. The rest of the year is dry. Temperatures vary, but on average do not go lower than 15° Celsius and range up to 26° or 30°. Adaptation to Canada's cold climate is therefore a problem for many Vietnamese immigrants.

POPULATION

In 1984 there were about sixty million people living in Vietnam with 80 per cent of them in rural areas engaged in farming rice, maize, soybeans, coffee, rubber, and tea. The urban population is mainly in three large cities, Hanoi, Ho Chi Minh City (formerly Saigon), and Haiphong. More than half the population is under sixteen. Life expectancy is sixty-seven years for women and sixty-three for men.

ETHNIC AND CULTURAL GROUPS IN VIETNAM

While the large majority of the population in Vietnam is Vietnamese, there are several minority ethnic groups. These include the Thai,

Muong, Tho, Cham and Kha (Malay-Indonesians), East Indians and, of most significance for migration to Canada, the Chinese, who comprise about 2 per cent of Vietnam's population. Traditionally, Vietnamese are farmers and fishermen but many now live in the cities and hold various kinds of jobs. All speak Vietnamese which varies only slightly across the country.

The Chinese have been in Vietnam for many generations, and came generally from south China. The majority speak Cantonese or Trieu Chan, a dialect of Buangdong province. Most of them, particularly those in southern Vietnam, run urban businesses, ranging from one-person food stalls to large import-export enterprises. The Chinese community remains separate from the Vietnamese, each having its own residential communities, schools, and organizations. Each, too, holds negative stereotypes about the other, a pattern that tends to persist after migration to Canada.

HISTORY OF VIETNAM

Vietnam has for many centuries struggled against outside powers interested in its rich farm lands and its strategic position. Up until the advent of the trade-hungry European powers in Asia in the 1600s, China sometimes occupied and controlled Vietnam. At other times China was repelled. However, European expansion brought first the Portuguese and, subsequently the French. The latter penetrated Vietnam by means of Catholic missions and the French East Indian Company. In 1883 Vietnam became a colony of France even though twenty years of military activity ensued before the Vietnamese were "pacified." Except for a period during the Second World War when the Japanese ruled and for a short-lived period of Vietnamese independence in 1945–46, French dominance continued until 1954. In that year the Vietnamese, led by Ho Chi Minh, the Communist party leader, defeated the French at the famous battle of Dien Bien Phu.

After this first Vietnam War an international agreement divided the country into North and South, with the Communist party in control of the North and the nationalist regime supported by the United States in charge of the South. The North, backed mainly by Russia, eventually won the second Vietnam War in 1975 when the American forces were withdrawn and the nationalist regime in the South was driven out. Since the fall of Saigon in 1975 the Communist party has unified the country which became known as the Socialist Republic of Vietnam in 1976.

These political upheavals have meant change in many aspects of

Vietnamese society. In particular, French rule led to the introduction of French language and culture, and Roman Catholicism, the building of cities, and land policies which changed the rural class structure; some rural farmers became rich landowners while others lost their land and became labourers. Large extended families began to break up so that only parents and the eldest son and his family lived together. Younger children meanwhile found homes elsewhere. More village people moved to towns and took low-level jobs while an enlarged urban middle class began to appear simultaneously. Thus "modernization" occurred in many aspects of Vietnamese life.

However, much more radical change occurred in the North after 1954 and in the whole country after 1976. To achieve the goal of destroying all social classes the government in the North took rigorous economic and political measures such as confiscating private property, collectivizing land, and nationalizing production. Individual liberties were abolished and men and women were judged to be equal. Polygamy and early marriages were prohibited and two classes were officially recognized; public service workers (teachers, factory workers, and so on) and peasants working on the land. Somewhat different policies were followed in the South where, since 1976, private business as well as co-operatives, communes, and other government-controlled systems were allowed.

Recent events in the country have meant that a large number of Vietnamese belonging to specific subgroups have left the country.

MIGRATION TO CANADA

There were about 1,000 Vietnamese living in Canada prior to the end of the Vietnam War. Most were students or professionals who had come for training or economic advancement, and settled in the east, particularly in Quebec, where their knowledge of French was helpful.

However, large numbers of people from Vietnam came to Canada later in two separate waves. The first immediately followed the end of the war in 1975–76, and the second larger wave began in 1978, and is still not fully completed. The first group, about 5,000 people, were mainly political refugees who had been associated with the South Vietnamese government or the American forces and whose lives would have been in danger after the Communist take-over. Many brought skills, language, and experiences which facilitated adaptation to Canada, since they tended to be middle class, urban, and relatively well-educated. Many left behind most of their property and often some family members.

The second, much larger wave of refugees was generally referred to as the "boat people" although not all of them escaped Vietnam in that way. As the Communist regime began to reorganize Vietnam's economy and society, an initial trickle of refugees began to appear in places like Malaysia, Thailand, and Hong Kong in 1978. But that trickle soon turned into a torrent; for example, it is estimated that in one month, June 1979, 57,000 people left Vietnam by boat. This enormous exodus was at least in part encouraged and approved by the Vietnamese government. Almost all of these migrants found themselves in refugee camps elsewhere in Asia or in the U.S., where they awaited admittance by Canada and other countries.

This second wave of immigrants from Vietnam to Canada amounted to more than 18,000 people in 1979 and more than 23,000 in 1980. While numbers have subsequently decreased, Vietnam still provides more refugees to Canada than any other country, at least up until 1985. Most of the recent arrivals are relatives of earlier refugees and are being reunited with their families.

People who left Vietnam after 1978 represent a much broader segment of the population than those who left earlier. Some of those who came to Canada were ethnic Vietnamese who had migrated from North to South Vietnam when the Communists took over the North in 1954; others were Northerners who went South later. However, a very large proportion of the refugees who came to Canada were ethnic Chinese who had lived in Vietnam for years, indeed generations. Their decision to leave was based partly on the Communist government's economic changes which resulted in Chinese-owned businesses being expropriated by the state and the relocation of the former owners to the countryside or to "new economic zones." Some Chinese left after the breakdown of diplomatic relations between Vietnam and the People's Republic of China. Loss of livelihood and traditional antagonism and distrust between Vietnamese and Chinese led the latter to fear for their future. Some fled across the northern border to China but most left by boat.

The experiences of the "boat people" were devastating. What property they were able to carry was often stolen or used to pay bribes before embarking. Once on the sea pirates preyed on the boats, raping and murdering for the sake of what they could steal. One estimate is that 50 per cent of those who left Vietnam's shores died or were murdered on the way. This experience has been reflected, in the West, in the mental health problems experienced by refugees from Vietnam.

Those who did survive the exodus were held in refugee camps in Malaysia, Hong Kong, Thailand, and Indonesia, asylum being offered reluctantly for fear of ethnic conflict and because of lack of support funds in those countries. The United Nations and other international agencies gave financial support, and systems for screening and accepting refugees were instituted. But for the refugees themselves, this resulted in delays of months and years before they were allowed to move on.

Once they arrived in Canada, Vietnamese refugees were initially aided by the federal government or by private sponsors, many of them church groups. The largest group of Vietnamese has settled in Quebec, mainly Montreal, although there are also significant numbers of Vietnamese in Alberta and BC, mostly in urban areas. Neither the ethnic Vietnamese immigrants nor the Chinese from Vietnam had forerunners in Canada whose community they could join. The Vietnamese distinguish themselves in terms of northern and southern origin, and along political and class lines. Thus they could not easily join the earlier arrivals. Chinese from Vietnam, even though they speak Cantonese, are not usually thought of as equals by the Hong Kong Chinese community. In contrast to many other immigrant groups the people from Vietnam were faced with the task of constructing their own sense of community and finding ways to survive.

JOBS AND INCOME IN CANADA

When the large wave of Vietnamese refugees arrived in Canada government and private sponsors provided initial financial aid, but both groups expected that refugees would quickly find jobs. Getting work was just as important to the refugees themselves who were keen to be financially independent. At the beginning most men were forced by necessity and lack of English to take low-level service and factory jobs that were often incompatible with their previous, higher levels of training, education, and work experience. To meet living expenses, and to buy clothing and medicines to send home to less fortunate relatives, many men took on two jobs, working very long hours for little pay. An additional incentive to take two jobs, to search for work before they had learned adequate English or to move to better-paying but perhaps dead-end jobs, was the need to document savings and earnings in order to sponsor further family migrations to Canada.

While it was not common for women to work outside the home in Vietnam, many immediately did so in Canada where a second income was necessary to meet living expenses. As with the men, women were largely limited to poorly paid jobs in factories, hotels, hospitals, and restaurants. As a result, by 1981, 59 per cent of adult

Southeast Asian women in Canada were working, a fact that entailed considerable change in family responsibilities and roles.

Initially, then, the refugees from Vietnam took whatever jobs they could get—often poorly paid and insecure—and frequently found two jobs in order to augment income. Many who arrived in 1979-80 have managed to obtain training, upgrade skills, improve English, and thus have moved into more stable and better paid employment. However, there are still Vietnamese who are overqualified for their jobs partly because they cannot afford to take time off work to obtain Canadian qualifications. There are many whose jobs are still insecure especially during economic recession; it was estimated that 30-40 per cent of Vietnamese lost their jobs in Alberta in 1981-82 when the economic downturn occurred. Thus, while Vietnamese are generally hard-working and eager to earn, they, like most immigrants, suffer by coming in at the bottom of the economic system where security and pay are low. The economic burden is even greater because many feel strong obligations to help relatives left at home or still in refugee camps.

RELIGION

As is true of several Asian cultures, people in Vietnam have a rather pluralistic view of religion. That is, a family might identify itself as Buddhist but might also worship at a variety of shrines and follow the precepts of Confucianism. Only the Christians, who comprise 10-15 per cent of Vietnam's population, and are mostly Roman Catholic, see themselves as belonging to a specific religious organization with a distinctly different set of practices. Even then, many recognize the values that are associated with the traditional religions.

For example, the majority of Vietnamese try to follow the central teachings of Confucius: to serve one's king or country; to respect one's teachers and father; to behave as a good and wise man. From Buddhism comes the idea of karma, which holds that one's destiny is determined in accordance with the virtue and vice of past lives. And pervasive throughout Vietnam is ancestor worship, whereby the souls of one's ancestors are believed to be the natural protectors of one's family. In Vietnamese homes in both Vietnam and Canada, there may be a small altar dedicated to Buddha and to family ancestors at which family members offer prayer and seek ancestral blessings.

Most Vietnamese who came to Canada are Buddhists, yet initially there were few Buddhist temples or organizations, similar to those at home, for them to join. Over the years, however, in places like Calgary and Edmonton, Vietnamese Buddhist Associations have been organized to provide places of worship and mutual support. Since Vietnamese are generally flexible about religious membership and since many were sponsored by Canadian Protestant groups, some Vietnamese participate in or organize their own Protestant churches, such as the Vietnamese Alliance Church in Vancouver.

LANGUAGE

In their home country, the majority group speaks Vietnamese and the Chinese minority usually speaks both Cantonese and Vietnamese. Those who had government, large business, and other professional jobs were likely to know French or English or both. Among Vietnamese speakers there are accent differences that make it difficult for northerners and southerners to understand those from the central area of the country.

While the earliest wave of immigrants from Vietnam usually had fluency in French and thus settled largely in Montreal, later waves had more mixed backgrounds and were less likely to speak either English or French. Some could not read or write their own spoken language, whether Vietnamese or Cantonese. Thus, for the largest proportion of people from Vietnam the language problem in Canada was acute.

When the first immigrants began to arrive, job placement was thought to be the solution to the language problem, since it was believed that English or French would be picked up easily at work. This seemed not to happen, particularly because adult men and women often took jobs in which little English was required, or because most of their fellow workers were also Vietnamese. Moreover, when refugees did attend English language classes, as most did, it was after long working hours. Even today, "the classes are filled with tired Indochinese, who, having worked all day and attended to the demands of their families, are struggling to learn a new language" (Indra 1985:457). In the meantime, the young children learn English or French quickly and become the go-betweens thus threatening the traditional authority of father and mother. The adult's sense of isolation and lack of control over individual and family life often continues for as long as he or she is not comfortable in the new language.

FAMILY STRUCTURE

For a person from Vietnam, the family is the main source of identity, and loyalty to family is primary. In Vietnam, the traditional family in the village often included elderly grandparents, an adult couple, and their unmarried children, along with married sons and daughters-in-law. While large and close families are still the ideal, nuclear families with husband, wife, and their children are now more common, given the socio-economic changes in modern Vietnam. Even though large family networks may not actually live in the same home, the authority of elders, especially male elders, is still recognized as is their right to be consulted when major family decisions are made, such as marriage or land purchase. The hierarchical family structure extends to all, for even older siblings have authority over younger and must be shown respect. In Canada, confusion sometimes results for Vietnamese children when two siblings of different ages are placed in the same grade at school, thus contradicting the customary hierarchical relationship.

Traditionally and currently in Vietnam women have fewer rights than men. For example, women currently have less access to education, fewer political opportunities, and receive less work points than men. However, Vietnamese women often have had the opportunity to work or earn money, and many belong to professional, middle-class urban families, or have run small businesses such as village rice mills. Indeed women are considered "more rational and calculating in financial matters than men" (van Esterisk 1980:160). Thus, in the family, while elder men must be approached for major decisions the wife or mother enjoys considerable power and independence, usually of a subtle variety.

Many families were separated when attempting to leave Vietnam, so that by the time refugees arrived in Canada they often had heart-rending stories to tell. Some had to leave the country alone, having been chosen by the family to use meagre family funds to go abroad, in the hope that others might follow later. Others describe becoming separated during the exodus or in the refugee camps and many still search for lost family members. In Canada many refugees initially created substitute "families," for economic and emotional reasons, by joining together with others to share a house or apartment. Some intact families took in those who had arrived alone creating "extended" families. Initially, then, it was unusual to find a single nuclear family living alone; few could afford it.

Obligations to family members outside Canada continue to be very strong, often limiting the individual's or family's ability to become established in Canada. A conflict arises between saving money to sponsor family members as immigrants or to make down payments on a house. There is also conflict between dropping a second job to make time for English classes or retaining two jobs to earn enough to send parcels to those still in refugee camps. While Vietnamese generally see themselves as long-term residents of Canada, their extended family, to whom they have great obligations, may be scattered throughout the world.

As is true of many immigrants, when people first arrive in Canada it is often easier for women to get jobs than for men. In many cases these women did not have paid work in Vietnam. These developments created considerable strain on the relationships between men and women. The man's authority and his role as the family bread-winner is undermined when his wife supports the family, and when more of the "women's work" is left to him. More strain develops if his wife seeks after the independence and equality she sees in relationships between Canadian couples. The fact that Vietnamese women often continue to work even after their husbands find jobs means that readjustments may continue far beyond the initial years in Canada.

As refugees from Vietnam have become more established in Canada and have moved beyond initial concerns about re-establishing families and providing basic economic security, other family issues become more important. Children learn English easily, quickly adapt to Canadian lifestyles, and begin to grow away from their families. These issues often create family conflict particularly at adolescence, and parents begin to feel that they are losing their hitherto unquestioned authority over their growing children. Adolescents may forget the Vietnamese language, or not want to use it, may openly question parental advice, or may even choose to move out of their parents' home once they have jobs. Parents often feel helpless when these conflicts begin to arise. They see children quickly losing the Vietnamese or Chinese culture that parents often want to preserve. Also, the questioning of parental advice by adolescent children often coincides with parental realization that the family's future rests, not with themselves, but with the children. Thus the valued culture is further jeopardized.

CHILD-REARING

From the point of view of Canadians, it may appear that Vietnamese families spoil their babies. Babies are usually not allowed to cry but instead are held by the mother or an older sibling who may talk or sing softly to the infant. One result of this practice is that Vietnamese children do not start walking as early as Western children. When a new baby absorbs all the mother's attention, the older child is often abruptly weaned and its care may be handed over to an older sibling. The child who raises his or her younger sibling may continue to have close lifelong relationships with that sibling.

Most child discipline and training is by example and thus is not usually a planned strategy. For example, toilet-training occurs when small children imitate their older siblings. In many families in Vietnam, toddlers may not wear diapers or underpants and urinate wherever they happen to be. The same learning by experience strategy is used for teaching other skills to young children: what to eat and wear, and how to speak. When parents do discipline their children it may be by speaking in a quiet manner, but also by shouting or slapping. Sometimes a child who has misbehaved may be asked to kneel facing the wall and to remain there for some time. Parents are believed to be within their rights to beat a child and outsiders are not expected to intervene, but such beating rarely occurs. However, Vietnamese parents do expect their children to follow their guidance without discussion or question. One result of this is that children do not usually express their anger openly but instead are more likely to be stubborn or passively unco-operative.

MARRIAGE

In Vietnam, in both Vietnamese and Chinese families, marriages are generally arranged by both sets of parents and it is rare for couples to make independent choices. Since families are traditionally structured along parental lines the new wife moves to her husband's father's home, thus joining a new family and learning to live and work with her mother-in-law. While most marriages are within each ethnic community, some Chinese men take Vietnamese wives.

Traditionally neither husband nor wife expects a marriage to be close and personally fulfilling. Husbands and wives tend to socialize separately and if the husband sometimes drinks or visits prostitutes with his friends, the wife will shrug the matter off as typical of male behaviour. The marriage itself is not usually threatened.

When the largest waves of people arrived in Canada from Vietnam there were many single men without families, fewer young unmarried women, and few intact families. The young men, once they had become economically established, at first often travelled long distances to find Vietnamese wives, and some married women from other Asian countries, such as the Philippines. There have been few intermarriages with white Canadians.

DIVORCE

As is true of many cultures in which marriages are arranged and thought of as family contracts, divorce is uncommon. Women usually choose to endure the marriage rather than to suffer ostracism for having left their husbands.

NAMES

Names of both Vietnamese and Chinese people from Vietnam are often confusing to record keepers although people often adapt their names to Western conventions after they have lived in Canada for a while. However, family and given names are traditionally put in the opposite order from Western names so that the family name comes first and the given name last, with one or sometimes two names in between. For example, a Chinese man might be named Wang Din Wah (comparable to Jones Tom Harry) or a Vietnamese man might be Nguyen Trong Thiet (comparable to Smith Jim George).

Women in both Chinese and Vietnamese communities usually do not change their names after marriage. Thus married couples do not have family names in common.

Common Chinese surnames from Vietnam are: Chau, Ha, Luu, Ly, Luong, Ong, Pho, Tang, Vyong. Those for Vietnamese are: Cao, Dinh, Hoang, Le, Luu, Ly, Ngo, Nguyen, Phan, Tran. Because at least two Vietnamese surnames are very common (Nguyen and Tran), Vietnamese people are commonly distinguished informally by use of their given name rather than their family name. For example, Nguyen Trong Thiet may be called "Mr. Thiet" in order to distinguish him from the many other people sharing the family name of Nguyen. Or a personal characteristic may be added (Vien map, or "fat Vien") to distinguish individuals.

AGES

In some instances confusion about a child's age may arise since, traditionally, a baby is one year old at birth, rather than at the end of the first year of life.

VALUES

Many people from Vietnam are preoccupied with maintaining face and avoiding open disagreement or confrontation. So long as relationships, particularly with one's superiors, are smooth everyone knows how to behave, and everyone knows who has obligations to whom. Thus it is important to smile and to agree even when neither action really means consent or agreement. A Canadian doctor may suspect that a Vietnamese patient has stopped taking prescribed medicines. However, the patient may deny the allegation, feeling that he should avoid embarrassing the physician by acknowledging that the doctor's orders have been disregarded. Public health nurses may expect that a mother will bring her child to a well-baby appointment to which she has apparently agreed only to find that the mother's so-called agreement was a polite "yes" meant to avoid disagreement, not to affirm the nurse's recommendation. To Westerners these actions may seem evasive, but to the person from Vietnam they are honourable, and are meant to prevent mutual embarrassment.

GESTURES

Facial expressions and body movements common to people from Vietnam are clearly related to their high valuation of smooth and predictable relationships. They prefer formal relationships with others, not the first name, sometimes joking or effusive mode of conversation adopted by Westerners. Politeness is important, resulting in smiles that do not necessarily mean agreement or even understanding. Impassive facial expressions and controlled body movements often make it difficult for Canadians to understand what a Vietnamese person is thinking. Yet, for the Vietnamese, this politeness and formality is entirely proper.

Vietnamese people are sometimes uncomfortable with steady and direct eye contact and would prefer fleeting glances. The person's head is believed to be sacred and therefore should not be touched without prior explanation. Thus patting a child on the head, a common gesture in the West, does not have the same meaning in Vietnam. Just as the head is sacred, the feet are profane and should not be pointed directly towards another person.

TRADITIONAL HEALTH BELIEFS AND PRACTICES

In pre-colonial times, Vietnamese used a variety of strategies to deal with illness: herbal remedies that helped the body regain equilibrium; isolation of the sick if the disease was communicable or highly stigmatized; and visits to shrines and temples if offerings to the gods could help cure. Even now when Western biomedical treatment is also available, traditional beliefs are common and traditional methods of treatment are often the family's first choice. Many of these beliefs have been brought to Canada and traditional methods continue to be used alongside, or instead of, Western biomedicine.

There are four main notions about illness in traditional Vietnamese medical beliefs and practices: hot and cold equilibrium; good and bad wind and water; supernatural causes of illness; and hereditary causes of illness.

Hot and Cold

This idea comes from Chinese medicine's concern with two opposing forces in the universe, yin and yang, represented in medicine as hot and cold. Heat and cold in the body must be in perfect equilibrium if illness is to be avoided. Where there is too much heat in the body fever, colitis, or skin eruptions may result. Excess cold explains fainting, common diarrhoea, or paralysis, among others. The delicate body balance can be upset in many ways, for example, by strong emotions. But the most important disturbance is from the foods one chooses to eat. Some foods are hot, others cold, so careful choice is required to retain, or regain, equilibrium. Some herbal medicines, also classified as hot or cold, aid in balancing the body.

Thus, according to these beliefs, a woman is in a cold condition after childbirth because she has lost heating blood. She should therefore avoid drinking cold juice or water and should not shower or wash her hair. If a person has fever there is concern that heat is being lost. Consequently, the feverish patient should be warmly covered, should avoid foods classified as cold (many vegetables and fruits), and should eat heating foods such as eggs and rice. Our Western pills, in fact all biomedicine, are believed to be hot and sometimes are not taken, or the dosage reduced, if the patient believes that the illness is a hot one.

Because many illnesses are believed to be the result of excess bodily heat or cold a person from Vietnam sometimes describes them as such, thereby confusing Canadian health professionals. For example, if a Vietnamese complains of being "hot," he does not necessarily have a fever but may have a symptom believed to be caused by an imbalance of heat in the body, such as constipation, dark urine, or hoarseness. A "weak heart" may refer to fainting, dizziness, or feelings of panic; a "weak kidney" to sexual dysfunction; and "weak nerves" to headaches or inability to concentrate.

Wind and Water

This notion too derives from Chinese medicine. The Vietnamese classifies wind (or air) and water as good or bad. A bad wind can act fast to induce high fever, convulsion, and even sudden death. Bad water is believed to have a slower effect on health, causing chronic fever, anaemia, or muscle wasting.

An attack of a bad wind is believed to require emergency measures to dispel it quickly. For some manifestations of bad wind (such as headache, cough, motion sickness), the bad wind can be released by creating small bruises on the body, commonly effected by rubbing the body with a coin or a spoon, or by cupping, that is, by placing a hot cup on the body and letting it cool until the air contracts and draws the skin upward. When bruise lines appear the bad wind has come to the surface and left the body. In some cases in Canada, health professionals have suspected child abuse when they discover these bruises on a child's body. In fact, parents have simply used a traditional medical treatment that is believed to help cure.

Supernatural Beliefs

Supernatural forces are often used to explain mental illness and, in the past, epidemics. A mentally ill person may have done something to offend a god who, in turn, punishes the individual by making him behave crazily. Or, his body may simply have been possessed by a ghost or demon who uses it to go about his devilish work. Ghost possession can be treated by a sorcerer who goes to the sick person's home and invokes Taoist deities to chase the ghost away. If this is not successful after repeated seances the mad person might be confined inside a Buddhist temple where the ghost will flee in fear of Buddha. Cure is believed to occur if the sick person stays long enough at the temple to ensure that the ghost forgets about him.

Prior to the arrival of biomedicine, with its immunizations and more effective treatment of communicable disease, epidemics were explained as an army draft from the occult world. This world mirrored Oriental society, with a king, mandarins, army, farmers, and so on. When the king needed soldiers he came to draft them from the people of Vietnam. The living victims were marked with skin eruptions that sometimes looked like the imprint of the army's stamp.

Heredity

Traditionally in Vietnam, many communicable diseases were

believed to be hereditary, a plausible belief since many members of the same family came down with the same illness, such as tuberculosis or leprosy.

Some family names became notorious for the diseases from which they suffered. And other families exhorted young people to choose carefully the family name and stock of the partner they wanted to marry in order to avoid such inherited diseases. Eligible young men and women from the unfortunate families had to travel to distant regions to seek marriage partners.

Many diseases believed to be inherited became highly stigmatized, particularly leprosy. Lepers lived alone in small huts outside the village fence, and had no contact with anyone. Food was left for them at the door.

More recently, with the advent of Western biomedicine in Viet nam, beliefs about hereditary illnesses accord much more closely with Western ones although some of the traditional "hereditary" diseases are still stigmatized, for example, leprosy.

TRADITIONAL MEDICAL PRACTITIONERS

As is true in most societies, Vietnamese usually try home remedies before going to a medical practitioner. But if the herbal concoctions or particular foods do not effect cure, the next step for many is a visit to a herbal practitioner. Some of these subscribe to a theory taught by Chinese-trained "professors" (northern herbalists) while others follow folk theory (southern herbalists). Each herbalist also owns a medicinal herb shop and may have inherited family formulas to treat specific diseases such as asthma, piles, or fractures, for example. While being treated by the herbalist, patients are usually less concerned with knowing the diagnosis than with obtaining appropriate medicines, usually taken in the form of dry ingredients. It is left to the family to cook the herbs carefully and to give the bitter infusion to the patient each day.

BIOMEDICINE IN VIETNAM

The French brought biomedicine to Vietnam in the last century but health services were slow in developing, particularly in rural areas. Some attempts were made to control epidemics through vaccination programs but not until Vietnamese themselves began to be trained as physicians did ordinary people in the towns begin to use biomedicine. People in rural areas continued to rely on herbal doctors and home remedies for most health care.

Before 1975, in South Vietnam, there was one doctor per 10,000 people. Currently the Vietnamese government reports that there is one physician for every 4,000 people (compared to Canada's one per 550) and these doctors are supplemented by "assistant doctors" who work in village health stations and refer some patients to district hospitals. Hospital care, where it is available, is now free except that patients must pay for their own food; it is common for families to bring food from home. Prior to 1975, hospitals provided food. Rural health services are more developed in the north than the south and there is a shortage of drugs and medical supplies. Until recently, at least, some biomedicines were sold by drugstores without prescription even though selling such medicines was illegal. Thus a family doctor practising in Vietnam during the 1960s and 1970s often saw patients with infections that were resistant to antibiotics, because many patients had used antibiotics at home in insufficient dosages, for short duration, and for inappropriate symptoms.

COMMON DISEASES IN VIETNAM

For the period before the arrival of Western biomedicine in Vietnam information about disease is sketchy, but it is clear that fertility rates were high and many babies died in the first year. The two killer diseases mainly responsible were gastroenteritis and pneumonia. Malaria, tuberculosis, smallpox epidemics, cholera, typhoid fever, plague, meningitis, and polio were also prevalent. Venereal diseases were not common since casual sex was taboo. Parasitical diseases such as tapeworm and hookworm were endemic and poverty explained high rates of malnutrition. Beriberi from vitamin B deficiency due to the low protein rice diet often resulted in cardiac complications or paralysis. Oedema was also common.

With the development of modern medicine and the expansion of preventative measures, many of these diseases have been eradicated, controlled, or effectively treated. The recent improvements in health are evident in the life expectancy of sixty years in 1980 and an infant mortality rate of 35 infant deaths per 1,000 births (compared to Canada's 10 per 1,000). Malaria is still endemic but better treatment and prevention are available. Tuberculosis is less prevalent and more easily cured. Leprosy is more adequately treated, and malnutrition has been reduced by better transportation, more even food distribution among the population, and also improved education and treatment.

DISEASES IN CANADA

Immigrants from Vietnam were and are relatively free of communicable diseases when they arrive in Canada because they have been medically screened abroad. Upon arrival there are sometimes other health problems apparent that can be treated fairly easily, for example, intestinal parasites and anaemia. Children are often incompletely immunized and some people suffer from malnutrition. The standard Harvard height and weight chart is not always useful in assessing malnutrition in children since Vietnamese body sizes are often small; a well nourished Vietnamese child may fall within the 3 to 10 percentile range. As is true for people from countries where medical services are limited, there may be genetically caused problems that have not been corrected such as extra fingers and toes.

There are, however, four major diseases that are sometimes brought to, or appear in, Canada among the Vietnamese people. Hepatitis B is prevalent in the refugee camps where water is often contaminated. In some cases as many as 20 per cent of a camp's population might contract the disease. As it is mostly in sub-clinical form, it will only become apparent if a positive antigen reaction is shown in a blood test. Hepatitis B vaccination is advisable for medical and dental staff working with people from Vietnam and for babies born of carrier mothers since it is contagious through blood-to-blood contact. At present it is not clear whether vaccination is necessary for the spouse or sex partner of the infected person.

Pulmonary tuberculosis is sometimes present in immigrants from Vietnam, usually in inactive form since tuberculosis screening is required for admission to Canada. If reactivation occurs, it is often during the first five years of the newcomer's stay in Canada. It is important for all those with inactive tuberculosis to make regular visits to TB control clinics for examination and treatment for at least five years.

Leprosy, found only in tuberculoid form in Vietnam, can be easily missed by a medical officer conducting the immigration screening examination because its signs and symptoms may be so minor as to be mistaken for trivial skin diseases if indeed they are spotted at all. Some cases have been discovered in Canada among refugees from Vietnam. Tuberculoid leprosy does not spread by casual contact and out-patient treatment is readily available from dermatologists. It is important to refer patients who present long lasting and hypo-aesthetic skin lesions.

Malaria is sometimes brought from Vietnam but cannot spread in

Canada because the parasite does not thrive outside the body and the anopheles mosquito carrier is absent. The disease is sometimes reactivated when the person has a low state of resistance, and gives rise to inexplicably high and protracted fever. Persons who do suffer a recurrence of malaria should be advised against donating blood.

After several years of residence in Canada, the immigrants from Vietnam generally present a good health picture. However, there is a tendency for them to develop certain specific diseases. Dental problems, both cavities and gum diseases, are common complaints. On coming to Canada some immigrants may take in less calcium if they live in soft water areas; moreover, they often eat softer foods than before, thereby depriving their teeth of the invigoration of chewing tougher vegetables. Dental visits are often delayed until there are several problems mainly because of the high cost of dental care in Canada.

Constipation and haemorrhoids are fairly common and are often linked. They are largely the result of a switch to softer foods with less dietary fiber. Some people drink insufficient fluid at work to avoid going to the bathroom during working hours.

Newcomers to Canada also catch viral diseases very easily since they are not immune to the local viruses. For example, they are highly susceptible to respiratory infections during the influenza season.

RELATIONSHIP BETWEEN DOCTOR AND PATIENT

As in the past, people in Vietnam still defer to health professionals. Doctors are special persons who are regarded as having a godsent gift to save the people and help society. The traditional high status of physicians was strongly reinforced when Western medicine was brought to the region by French doctors who were also respected and awe inspiring government employees. Physicians are expected to be wise, to have good judgement, and to be dignified and Vietnamese patients entrust almost total responsibility for medical decisions to the doctor. For the average person in Vietnam, the health professional is consequently rather remote and aloof.

Consistent with the hierarchical class structure in the society, the medical professions are also organized hierarchically. Nurses are perceived only as accessories to physicians, and their role is to carry out the doctor's orders, not to initiate activities, except when the doctor is absent. Nurses apply bandages, dispense pills, and give injections. A special position is reserved for public health nurses because they are government servants. As such they are respected and obeyed.

When they first go to a physician in Canada, people from Vietnam expect and prefer them to behave like those at home. The doctor should be formal and unhurried and patients assume that the physician in his wisdom will identify the illness without too many questions or an elaborate physical examination. Detailed questions about their lives, their past, or their families are particularly unwelcome especially if the patient can discern no connection between the questions and the illness. One patient complained that "Dr. Smith asked too many questions. I had the impression I was being examined by the Secret Police." Also, the very act of talking too much about an illness may indeed induce it, according to some people from Vietnam. Patients do not expect detailed explanation of the diagnosis nor the purpose of the recommended treatment. In fact, many people from Vietnam are unable to provide medical histories because their previous physicians did not generally inform them about such matters. However, the longer Vietnamese live in Canada the more they will tend to expect and require the physician to take a thorough history, perform a physical examination and ask detailed questions. In short, their expectations will increasingly conform to those of Westerners.

On the basis of past experience and customary preference, the Vietnamese patient will dislike removing more clothing than is absolutely necessary for a physical examination. In general, he prefers that touching of the body be kept to a minimum. For example, a patient who has a respiratory problem may only open the top of his shirt to allow the physician to listen to his chest.

Physicians are expected to inform the patient's family, who often accompany the patient, about the illness and treatment since other family members, particularly elders, often take responsibility for decisions and treatment.

Many Vietnamese prefer physicians from Vietnam even though they may be reticent about their past lives until they have established where the physician stood in Vietnam's complex political world. Many people from Vietnam choose Asian physicians where no Vietnamese doctors exist. They feel greater affinity even where the physician cannot speak Vietnamese. For gynaecological examinations, married women prefer female physicians and will accept a female nurse in the examining room, but not usually a family member. Unmarried women often are extremely reluctant to have pelvic examinations unless they are absolutely necessary and clearly explained.

Physicians are expected to take full command in accordance with their position and expertise, while patients from Vietnam expect to be passive and dependent. In Canada, health professionals may regard them as good patients because they ask few questions, make few complaints, and seem to comply with recommendations. To the Vietnamese this behaviour is felt to be polite, respectful to the professional, and protective of one's self, and thus generally helpful in avoiding embarrassment. The Vietnamese person will show respect to the professional by persistently addressing him as "Doctor." Politeness may mask misunderstanding and disagreement which may mean in turn that the patient sometimes disregards treatment recommendations and subsequent appointments.

Because physicians are held responsible for treatment and cure, many patients from Vietnam find recommendations to change their own behaviour (for example, by stopping smoking and changing diet) unacceptable or difficult to follow. Further, since they invariably expect doctors to prescribe medicines, other "natural" treatments that involve habit changes are less acceptable. For example, it would be very difficult to convince Miss Nguyen that she can use fluids and natural fibres in her diet to relieve constipation when laxatives can be prescribed by the physician.

Vietnamese people also tend to be quite stoical in the face of illness and pain. Men, in particular, are reluctant to reveal symptoms and sometimes delay treatment until pain or disability is great. This phenomenon is linked to beliefs about correct behaviour but also stems from the fact that many Vietnamese are paid by the hour and lose wages when attending appointments.

People from Vietnam often find it difficult to adapt to the Canadian physician's appointment system, and often tend to arrive late, at least initially. At home they were used to an entirely different system, whereby they dropped in at the office and waited their turn, or appeared at the beginning of the physician's office hours, took a number, and returned at the appropriate time later on.

HOSPITALS

In the past in Vietnam, a decision to go to hospital was made only when there was no other choice, for emergencies, when the patient's family could no longer provide care, or when all other treatments had failed. Hospitals were places to die. Although modern Vietnam has a much more satisfactory hospital system, many of the old beliefs and practices have not disappeared. Admission to hospital may be delayed beyond the optimal time for treatment; a patient may be taken home as soon as he appears to have improved; elderly patients in particular may avoid hospitalization or return home early to avoid dying in hospital.

While the patient is in a Vietnamese hospital, a family member usually stays with him or her to help nursing staff and to provide personal care. The family sends food from home so that the patient does not have to eat hospital food. In fact, in the Vietnamese language, to take care of a hospitalized patient is literally "to feed a patient." Many family members visit the patient at all times except at night or during physicians' rounds. Thus the family has considerable control over what is done for the patient and even what decisions are made about his treatment.

When a person from Vietnam goes to a Canadian hospital, some of the experiences from the past conflict with the Western hospital practices. In particular, older people are reluctant to be admitted to hospital because of its association with death. To die away from home is believed to bring bad luck on one's children and grandchildren and to confuse one's soul which may get lost on the way home or on its journey to Nirvana.

Although Vietnamese willingly share hospital rooms with others they prefer privacy and often want curtains pulled around the bed. Lack of privacy and fear of being overheard sometimes lead to evasive replies in answer to the doctor's questions. Problems of privacy are also posed by standard hospital gowns. Many people from Vietnam never reveal the body area between waist and knees, even to their closest relatives. They will wear hospital gowns if told to do so, but often with considerable embarrassment.

Because of traditional beliefs in the harmful effects of wind many Vietnamese show great concern about drafts in hospital rooms. They fear that a wind may aggravate serious illness and thus prefer to have windows closed at all times.

More subtle problems confront the family of a hospitalized person in Canada. In contrast with Vietnam, here the family can do very little for the hospitalized person. Food is provided by the hospital and additional foods from home are discouraged or forbidden. Visiting hours are limited and family nursing care is neither needed nor allowed. As a result, some families may feel that they have been forced to abandon the sick person.

MEDICINE AND OTHER TREATMENT

In Vietnam most people try home remedies first, before seeking a physician. Some of these remedies consist of herbal drinks designed to rebalance the body by cooling or heating. Very commonly used is a mentholatum-based ointment—Tiger Balm is an example—that is rubbed on the affected part of the body, inhaled, or swallowed to prevent or treat a wind disease.

Western-style biomedicines are also used at home, because in Vietnam many drugs are sold over the counter without prescription. Vietnamese families became aware of antibiotics, penicillin, and psychoactive drugs, for example, without learning of possible toxic effects or problems of resistance. Chloramphenicol which was introduced to treat typhoid fever became popular for all feverish diseases. There was no recognition that over-use could cause aplastic anaemia. In rare cases, families from Vietnam have brought chloramphenicol to the West for use at home.

If home remedies do not work, the Vietnamese patient goes to a doctor. In Vietnam, it was expected that a good doctor would give medicine and most physicians complied by prescribing not just one but several types of pills and perhaps one or more injections. For a patient it was unthinkable that no medicine would be given. Initially, in Canada, the same is expected of doctors. If the doctor says, "No medicine is really needed," a Vietnamese patient may feel cheated or misunderstood. Since patients expect rapid cures, a physician who repeats the same medication may find that the patient does not take it or fails to return; why should one continue with a medicine that does not work at once? Some may request certain drugs as they did in Vietnam, particularly "liver medicine" if there is digestive trouble or skin disease or "heart tonic" for weakness or dizziness.

While most people in Vietnam have used Western-style medicines, most of them purchased without prescription, there is still some resistance to their use. Biomedicine is believed to be hot and is thus felt to be risky if applied to hot conditions like fever. Also most people believe that Western medicines are too strong or inappropriate for Vietnamese. One way to avoid problems is to reduce the recommended dosage of biomedicines, a common practice among Vietnamese in Canada. Since some believe that Western biomedicines do not really apply to Vietnamese there is a tendency to stop taking medicines prematurely. Thus it is difficult to convince a patient that long-term medical treatment is beneficial, particularly where there are no evident symptoms, such as in cases of tuberculosis, high blood pressure, or diabetes.

Experiences with medical treatment as well as cultural beliefs in Vietnam lead Vietnamese to place high value on some Canadian medical procedures while attempting to avoid others. There is enthusiasm for injections, which may derive in part from past experiences with quick cures from penicillin injections, for example. People often insist on X-rays as well. Most laboratory tests are acceptable, such as urinalysis. However, many Vietnamese fear and resist blood tests that require even small samples of blood, mainly because they believe that the body has a finite, irreplaceable amount of blood. Some may attribute symptoms such as headaches or weakness to the loss of blood during blood tests, even single tests done several years earlier. Anti-pain medication is seldom requested probably because of the cultural value placed on stoicism.

Many health professionals in the West can attest to the reluctance of Vietnamese immigrants to agree to surgery. Only if they are convinced that there is no alternative will surgery be acceptable. Fear of surgery is probably explicable in terms of the earlier view that hospitals in Vietnam were places to die. However, resistance to surgery is also rooted in cultural belief, since the soul is believed to be attached to parts of the body. If those parts are removed or if the body is merely cut the soul might escape and death might ensue. Wandering souls are problematic for both the dead and the bereaved family. Especially in cases of minor surgery, for example, correcting strabismus, removing extra fingers and toes, Vietnamese may be particularly reluctant to consent. If they do, they may want to consult a horoscope to select an auspicious day.

CONTRACEPTION

Traditionally in Vietnam contraception was neither highly valued nor legal. The family was a source of happiness and children were highly appreciated. Furthermore, the French colonial authorities followed dominant Roman Catholic policy and discouraged modern birth control. Some herbal decoctions were used to prevent contraception or to induce abortion, but until recently most Vietnamese did not know about or use modern contraceptives.

Modern contraception was available in many refugee camps, however. Some women were given Depo-Provera, a long-term contraceptive injection, the serious side-effects of which have led to it being banned in Canada and the U.S. Some Vietnamese women in Canada request Depo-Provera while others are reluctant to use any contraceptive because of their bad experiences with Depo-Provera. However, having moved to the West where there may be no extended family to help and where rearing children is expensive, most women are willing to discuss modern contraception, particularly if the physician or nurse is a woman, and to accept some form of it.

PREGNANCY

Pregnancy is traditionally believed to be a normal condition, but one in which care should be taken to maintain the body's equilibrium. Thus pregnant women pay attention to the food they eat, and avoid too much hot food (for example, meat, alcohol, coffee) as well as cold food (for example, bananas). They may, however, crave foods that are astringent such as green mangoes. Tonics of various kinds are often taken, not only to strengthen the mother but to shrink the fetus so as to ease delivery. There is a strong belief that continued physical activity is important right up to the time of delivery. For this reason pregnant women often avoid naps or rest.

Not only are delivery and the physical health of the mother and child affected by behaviour during pregnancy, but so is the child's moral development. Pregnant women should avoid contact with people who are dishonest for fear of contaminating the unborn child. Moreover, the mother should behave impeccably herself by giving food to the poor, not complaining or being jealous, and so on. For similar reasons, sexual intercourse is ended at the third month of pregnancy.

More recently in Vietnam, formal prenatal care has been used by women, especially city dwellers. Thus some immigrants to Canada have had experience of regular check-ups and health education. Once in Canada, most women are willing to make regular prenatal visits to the physician and even attend prenatal classes, particularly where classes are conducted in Vietnamese or Cantonese. Some husbands are willing to attend as well.

CHILDBIRTH

The birth of a baby is a normal process. Vietnamese say, "The bud opens and the flower blooms." While many women who lived in urban Vietnam have had hospital deliveries by a physician, those from rural areas are more likely to have had babies at home with the help of a midwife. In both cases, women endured the pain of childbirth with stoicism and seldom with the benefit of an anaesthetic. Once in Canada, some of these practices begin to change, including the use of anaesthetics. If pain relief methods are made available, Vietnamese women use them and even request them, although the maintenance of self-control and stoicism during labour is still evident.

There is a tendency for infants born of women from Vietnam to weigh less at birth than Caucasian infants; the median weight for Vietnamese babies in one part of the U.S. was 3,260 grams as compared to 3,459 grams for Caucasians. However, the longer the family has stayed in the U.S. the more likely it is that birth weights approach the American norm.

All babies, whether male or female, are treated with tenderness. However, sons are preferred, as suggested by a common saying, "A single boy, that is positive; ten girls, that is still negative." Sons are important because they perpetuate the family name and allow the family to fulfil its responsibilities to the ancestors. Traditional methods were available that were thought to guarantee the sex of the child, such as planning conception on an odd-numbered day of the week in order to produce a son.

After childbirth, traditional medical beliefs classify the woman's body as cold because she has suffered stress and loss of blood during delivery. In rural Vietnam, therefore, many women followed the practices of "mother-roasting" common in Southeast Asia; that is, placing a small charcoal fire under the mother's bed to keep her warm. This practice has disappeared among urban women, but there are other ways of countering the cold imbalance, many of which are brought to Canada.

After birth, women are reluctant to bathe or wash their hair, for fear of cooling the body further. Instead, sponge baths with very warm water are much more acceptable. It is important, too, to avoid cold foods such as water, fruit juices, raw vegetables, and fruit. Hot, spicey, and salty foods are preferred, along with rice, eggs, tea, sweets, chicken broth, and a special "stew" made of rice, pork, and fish sauce. Avoiding drafts, air conditioning, and open windows is important. After birth the new mother expects and hopes to rest for at least one month.

Even in Canada, the one month period of rest is the ideal. If possible the new mother's own mother or her mother-in-law will come to help. The end of the baby's first month is celebrated by as large a party as the family can afford, for example, a backyard barbecue for as many as 150 guests.

In Vietnam's villages women commonly breast-feed for one-and-a-half years and usually let the child wean itself. Urban women, especially those who work, are more likely to bottle-feed. Babies are not usually offered solid food until six months. In Canada, despite the advocacy of breast-feeding by physicians and public health nurses, some women prefer bottle-feeding because it is more "modern," and others stop breast-feeding early because of conflict with jobs.

Babies and children who came to Canada from refugee camps were immunized before departing, and parents were told that immunizations were complete. This has created some confusion in Canada where additional immunizations for mumps and rubella are required. Careful explanations are needed before Vietnamese parents accept further immunizations.

MENTAL HEALTH

To people in Vietnam, mental illness usually means severe disorders, not the relatively minor problems such as depression or anxiety that Westerners often include in that category. Once a person becomes mentally ill there is little likelihood of cure. Mentally ill people are feared and rejected and their family members feel shame. It becomes the collective responsibility of the family to care for the sick person as long as his or her behaviour can be managed at home.

Traditionally, mental illness is often explained in astrological terms, such as being born under an unlucky star. Some suffer because of misdeeds in previous lives or the misdeeds of parents or ancestors. Malevolent spirits are also cited as causes. Treatments consist of exorcism ceremonies, rituals by Buddhist priests, and sometimes a stay at the Buddhist temple which is safe from demons. Meanwhile, family members devote themselves to good behaviour and religious piety.

After Western biomedicine came to Vietnam psychiatric hospitals became available, but only patients who were unmanageable and profoundly disturbed were taken there. The one large hospital, with 1,900 beds, provided little therapeutic activity for patients, few professional staff, and offered only electric shock and, later, drug therapy. Few expected the patient to return home. The psychiatric hospital was there to control the patient and indeed the majority of the staff were called "wardens." With the advent of psychotropic drugs some families began to seek biomedical treatment for a mentally ill member in the earlier stages of the illness, but most people adhered to traditional beliefs about causes and cures.

The experience of leaving home in Vietnam and eventually settling in Canada has certainly increased the risk of mental illness among these immigrants. The continuous war in Vietnam since 1945 has meant extensive dislocation of families within the country. Some of these internal refugees then left Vietnam in 1975 and with very little preparation. Many suffered terribly in the escape by sea. This was followed by prolonged stays in overcrowded and insanitary refugee camps. Upon arrival in Canada, some were settled in areas with no ethnic support groups, and where the climate was harsh. Many did not choose to leave their country. They have lost their homeland, and often their property, business, and customary social networks. Along with these losses have gone a lost sense of security, self-identity, and self-esteem. Separation from family is a major factor causing depression and anxiety. Some of these problems have been eased by subsequent reunion with family members and also by regrouping within Canada by means of moves from small towns to large metropolitan areas.

While many Vietnamese refugees manage to adjust to the new situation within three years or so, some have failed, particularly those who came with high hopes and unrealistic expectations. For many, there is still the nostalgia for the old country, guilt over leaving friends and family members behind, and a sense of being alien in the new homeland.

Some people from Vietnam do not manage to adjust to loss and change, and this may result in mental disturbance. Often these mental conditions are delayed reactions to loss and trauma, occurring six months to three years after arrival in Canada and precipitated by job loss, an automobile accident, or family conflict. Because families are ashamed and mental illnesses stigmatized, the sick person is often kept at home without treatment. First contact with formal treatment is sometimes in hospital emergency rooms, the sick person generally having arrived by police car or ambulance.

Families are reluctant to agree that minor psychiatric problems, such as adolescent problems in school, should be treated by a physician, particularly a psychiatrist. Consulting a psychiatrist is equivalent to declaring a family member insane.

Quite often, after a first contact with a psychiatrist or mental health clinic, the person resists all further treatment until he becomes ill or disturbed again. Only then is it possible for him to accept treatment, particularly if the professional has been able to establish a supportive mood and sense of trust in the very first encounter.

The culture of Buddhism stresses that "life is a sea of suffering" and that one should learn to cope with the individual stresses of daily life without burdening others with one's problems. Also, the Confucian social code teaches children to respect and obey teachers, parents, extended family members, and older siblings. Therefore, most psychiatric patients from Vietnam are not willing to discuss personal feelings about family or other more senior persons and almost all of them will describe their childhood as satisfactory. Thus, "talk therapy" that investigates family relationships and is used as the sole psychiatric treatment is unacceptable.

Instead, the patient and his family expect the mental health professional to establish what is wrong after only a brief history is taken, to make a diagnosis, and to provide medical treatment. A physical examination is expected; without it the psychiatrist is not a "doctor." Patients and their families are unfamiliar with and threatened by open-ended questions such as "Tell me about yourself" or "I wonder what you think of your illness." Moreover, a doctor who says, "I hope that we can work together in finding a solution" is not respected. Vietnamese expect the mental health professional to be authoritative and direct; they will accept and follow recommendations faithfully.

Thus, any kind of discussion of past experiences or current life problems is more acceptable if it is combined with medical treatment such as drug therapy, or with some kind of social intervention. Once the Vietnamese patient feels comfortable talking, it is useful to focus on psychosocial factors that may have contributed to the illness by discussing: (1) life, problems, and stresses in the home country; (2) escape or departure, who came, who stayed, the experience; (3) refugee camp experience; (4) attitudes towards and problems of being in Canada; (5) current worries and outlook for the future. These topics provide a framework for linking past experiences and current symptoms in ways the patient can understand, and in ways he may not have recognized before.

NUTRITION, FOOD, AND ALCOHOL

While French cuisine is popular among upper-class urban people in Vietnam, the vast majority of people prefer a diet in which boiled white rice is the staple. In fact, the literal translation of the word for "meal" is "time to eat rice." "A meal without rice is not a meal." In addition to rice, fresh green vegetables and fresh or dried fish are commonly served along with fermented fish sauce. If the family can afford it, chicken or pork in small quantities are also eaten. Noodles are sometimes substituted for rice, especially in soups. Water or tea are common beverages, and fruit is often eaten as a snack. The fat content of the traditional diet is low and normal calorific intake is about two-thirds of the Western norm.

Foods are classified as hot, cold, or neutral and it is important to balance these qualities so as to prevent illness. Thus the hot foods such as meat, fish sauce, sweets, coffee, spices, garlic, ginger, and onion should be offset by cold foods, for example, most vegetables, fruit, potatoes, fish, and duck. It is believed that many illnesses result from heat loss. If this happens, one should avoid cold foods. Common foods for people who are ill are a rice gruel to which sugar or sweetened condensed milk has been added or a dish made from pieces of salty pork with fish sauce.

In Vietnam, generally the same kinds of foods are served at all three meals. Rice along with vegetables and perhaps some meat are set out in bowls from which each person, including the young child, chooses what he or she wants. The family meal in which everyone sits together and where one course follows another is not common in Vietnam. Neither are meals occasions for conversation.

While rice wine is readily available in Vietnam, men do not consume large quantities of alcohol and women do not drink at all. When alcohol is used by men it is almost always during collective celebrations such as weddings. Lone drinking is rare. The value placed on formality, politeness, and face means that drunkenness is unacceptable. Also, as is true of other Asians, many people in Vietnam suffer uncomfortable physiological symptoms after consuming alcohol. Flushed faces, trembling, palpitations, and rapid breathing are common.

Generally, when people from Vietnam settle in Canada they prefer the foods that they ate in Vietnam, such as cha gio (deep-fried rice paper rolls filled with meat, egg, or chopped vegetables), pho (a soup made of noodles and meat), and nuoc man (fermented fish sauce). In urban areas many of these ingredients are available in Chinese markets. However, over the years some changes have occurred, in part because women who are employed do not have the necessary time to cook and also because many, particularly children, have developed a taste for Western foods.

Quick and relatively inexpensive fast foods have become popular, leading to a significantly increased consumption of soft drinks, peanut butter, ice cream, and pastries. While the diet of rice, fish, and vegetables is still the most common, many now eat significantly more milk, beef, butter, margarine, eggs, and potatoes. An increase in carbohydrates, sugar, and fat has meant that some Vietnamese, including children, have gained weight and a few have become obese. There is some evidence, too, that the nutritious, well-balanced Vietnamese diet has been replaced by a poorly balanced one.

A large proportion of Vietnamese, like many Asians, are intolerant of lactose, the sugar in milk. Using too much milk therefore produces diarrhoea and stomach-aches, mainly in those over age six.

Initially, refugees from Vietnam in Canada follow traditional drinking patterns; few men and no women drink. However, at least in some parts of the west, there has been an increase in alcohol use among men, particularly among the young, unmarried men who tend to drink in social groups. Scattered cases of alcoholism have been reported.

BATHING AND ELIMINATION

While daily bathing is important to people from Vietnam, there are some times when this is thought to be rather risky, mainly because bathing may cool the body and create illness. Therefore, a menstruating woman usually does not bathe or wash her hair, and the same prohibition applies after childbirth. If bathing is unavoidable during these risky times, a sponge bath with very hot water is thought to be safest.

In rural Vietnam, toilets are designed so that the individual can squat rather than sit, and flush toilets are rare. Initially, new immigrants to the West have some difficulty in adapting to the Western style of elimination.

DENTAL HEALTH

In Vietnam, there is approximately one dentist for every 40,000 persons compared to Canada's one per 2,175 people. As a result, only the very rich and privileged have had access to dental care. Lack of care, along with malnutrition and unbalanced diets because of protracted war in Vietnam and stays in refugee camps, has meant that many immigrants from Vietnam arrive in the West with serious dental problems. Both among adults and children there is a high incidence of missing and decayed teeth. For example, in one school in the U.S., 75 per cent of the Vietnamese children were in need of immediate dental care. Periodontal disease, indicated by spongy and bleeding gums, is also common.

Even though great value is placed on healthy white teeth and most Vietnamese are eager to receive dental care, a visit to a dentist in Canada may be postponed if money is needed for other more important priorities.

REHABILITATION

In Vietnam, very few medical resources were available for the rehabilitation of disabled people, for correction of birth defects, or for treatment of chronic diseases like epilepsy. Thus, immigrants to Canada do not have experience or knowledge of such efforts, and they often are uninterested in local rehabilitation programs. For example, braces for child victims of polio epidemics in Vietnam may not be accepted because the family feels that further suffering will result from additional medical attention. The need for long-term medication when there are no symptoms and little discomfort may not be understood by the family and medication may thus be stopped. Particularly in instances where surgical corrections are recommended, the Vietnamese decision-makers may feel that the dangers of surgery outweigh the benefits. They may therefore decide that it is better to live with, for example, strabismus or a cleft palate.

AGEING

Traditionally, old people in Vietnam were respected and privileged. Their long lives gave them the wisdom to advise the young and they were called upon when important decisions had to be made. Even after death they were respected and worshipped. All of the old persons' children were expected to return the parental concern and love they had received, but it was usually the eldest son who cared for parents in his home until their death.

Immigrants from Vietnam have generally been younger people, although as part of the more recent family reunification program, older people have begun to arrive. Many of the problems elderly people will experience have not yet occurred although some are probably predictable. With many husbands and wives at work, elderly parents, if they live in the same home, are likely to become baby-sitters and housekeepers, and will be isolated from the rest of the Vietnamese community. Also, their wisdom, probably very useful in Vietnam, may be less valuable in Canada where knowledge of local ways is crucial. Economic pressures may make the care of an ill or disabled parent at home extremely difficult. In the long run, veneration of the elderly as well as obligations to care may change. The quandary is well stated by an elderly Vietnamese in Canada. "You cannot send your father to an old-age home and then worship him after he dies" (Nguyen Quy Bong 1980:253).

DEATH AND DYING

Among the Vietnamese there is a very strong feeling that death should occur at home, not in hospital. At home one's family can provide comfort and one can die in peace. For some, death away from home means that the soul will wander, having no place to rest. Even for non-believers, death away from home is terrible. Often when a person is dying, the family will make every effort to take him or her home. If death does occur in a hospital it is important to move the body home as soon as possible.

Generally, the dying person's family wishes to be informed that death is imminent, but prefers that the patient himself should not be told. After death, families seldom, if ever, give permission for an autopsy unless it is required by law. Why cause more suffering to the dead person?

Traditional mourning practices entail family members wearing white clothing for fourteen days, followed afterwards by the wearing of black armbands. On the forty-ninth day after death the surviving family members organize a ceremony and food is provided for the entire family and those friends and neighbours who had given help. A smaller ceremonial gathering may occur after 100 days. Then, the person's eldest son organizes a ceremony each year on the anniversary of the death. The child or wife of the deceased person must wait three years to marry, and the husband must wait one year.

FURTHER READING

Bong, Nguyen Quy. "The Vietnamese in Canada: Some Settlement Problems," in K.V. Ujimoto and Grodon Hirabayeshi, eds., *Visible Minorities and Multiculturalism: Asians in Canada*. Toronto: Butterworth 1985

Chan, Kwok B. and Doreen M. Indra, eds. *Uprooting, Loss and Adaptation: The Resettlement of Indochinese Refugees in Canada*. Ottawa: Canadian Public Health Association 1987

Indra, Doreen. "Khmer, Lao, Vietnamese and Vietnamese-Chinese in Alberta," in Howard Palmer and Tamara Palmer, eds., *Peoples of Alberta: Portraits of Cultural Diversity*. Saskatoon: Western Producer Prairie Books 1985

Tepper, Elliot, ed. *Southeast Asian Exodus: From Tradition to Resettlement*. Ottawa: Canadian Asian Studies Association 1980

Muecke, Marjorie A. "In Search of Healers: Southeast Asian Refugees in the American Health Care System," *Western Journal of Medicine*, Vol. 139 (1983):835–40

Nguyen, San Duy. "Psychiatric and Psychomatic Problems among

Southeast Asian Refugees," *Psychiatric Journal of the University of Ottawa*, Vol. 7, No. 3 (1982):163-72

Tung, Tranh Minh. *Indochinese Patients: Cultural Aspects of the Medical and Psychiatric Care of Indochinese Refugees*. Washington, DC: Action for South East Asians 1980

Van Esterisk, P. "Cultural Factors Affecting the Adjustment of Southeast Asian Refugees," in *Southeast Asian Exodus: From Tradition to Resettlement*, Elliot Tepper, ed., pp. 151-72. Ottawa: Canadian Asian Studies Association 1980

CONTRIBUTORS

Donna Schareski (Vancouver City Health Department)
Vien Thien (MOSAIC, Vancouver)
Tammy Thiet (Vancouver City Health Department)

CHAPTER NINE

The West Indians

Joseph H. Glasgow and Eleanor J. Adaskin

There are people in Canada from nearly every island in the West Indies, but the majority living in western Canada are from Trinidad and Tobago, Jamaica, and Barbados. For this reason the material presented here will be confined mainly to people from those areas. Health professionals must recognize the diversity that exists among and even within islands, depending on socio-economic class and rural or urban setting, and note that the information presented here will describe some but not all West Indians in western Canada.

The material was gathered in 1986-7 by interviewing a small group of West Indians living in Winnipeg, and was subsequently validated with a larger group of Winnipeg West Indians. Differences are acknowledged among all West Indian individuals and communities, but it is hoped that health care professionals can benefit from knowing about some of the similarities.

GEOGRAPHY

The archipelago which constitutes the West Indian islands extends in the form of a crescent from the coast of Florida in North America to within seven miles of Venezuela in South America, and encloses a portion of the ocean which is divided into the Gulf of Mexico and the Caribbean Sea. There are forty large islands, some of which are little more than rocks. The total area of the West Indian islands is only 100,000 square miles, of which the British area, to which Trinidad and Tobago, Jamaica, Barbados belong, is slightly more than 12,000 square miles. The non-British West Indies are occupied by those who speak French, Spanish, and other languages, in addition to English.

HISTORY

The history of the West Indies clearly accounts for the variety of cultures that can be found there today and for the variety of immigrants who have come to Canada. In the early days some of the islands were captured and recaptured by the French, English, Spanish, and Dutch, hence the great diversity of people settling in the West Indies. Additional cultural groups were brought from Africa as slaves and, later, poor farmers from Scotland and Ireland, India, and China arrived to work on plantations.

In 1838, when slavery was abolished in the West Indies, many plantation owners became bankrupt. The government took over their estates and resold them, creating new opportunities for freed slaves and other poor immigrants to become paid workers in a growing variety of rural and urban jobs. Today, despite the strong American influences felt by most West Indians through television, trade, education, and tourism, historical and cultural traditions continue to exert an influence on West Indian communities whether they exist in the islands or have long since relocated to places such as Canada.

ECONOMY

The economy of the smaller West Indian islands is based mostly on cocoa, coffee, coconuts, citrus fruits, bananas, sugar cane, jams, jellies, condiments, and the tourist trade. In Jamaica and Trinidad there has been rapid expansion in manufacturing in a wide range of goods including textiles, tobacco, cement, plastics, and many food products. Jamaica is the world's leading producer of bauxite, while Trinidad is famous for its oils and asphalt and Barbados for its sugar and rum.

Despite the strong presence of foreign manufacturing companies in the West Indies, local governments are the major employers on many of the islands. However, unemployment remains a difficult problem, and serves as a major motive for emigration to countries such as Canada where jobs, education, and training options are more numerous and accessible. For a large proportion of the West Indians who have come to western Canada, university education has enabled them to occupy well-paid professional, managerial, and civil service positions. A smaller proportion of the West Indians in western Canada are in blue-collar and unskilled occupations such as construction, factory, or domestic work.

PEOPLE

Jamaica's motto, "Out of many, one people," points to the goal of valuing race and colour differences in an enriched and unified nation. The multicultural West Indian population is a rich mixture of people drawn from Africa, Asia, and Europe. Afro-Caribbeans, East Indians (Indo-Caribbeans), Chinese, Spanish, Portuguese, French, and British are very prominent in the islands. As well, there is a diminishing number of indigenous Carib Indians. Representatives of all of these groups or mixtures of groups constitute the West Indian immigrant population in Canada.

In the West Indies, as elsewhere, class distinctions exist, and are determined mainly by degree of affluence, education, and affiliation to those in authority. Colour in itself is no longer a significant barrier to advancement, since most leadership and professional positions in the West Indies are held by West Indians themselves, though this was not the case prior to the late 1960s. However, in Canada, despite the achievement of education, affluence, or powerful connections, West Indian people may encounter racial barriers whereby they are relegated to second class status on the basis of colour alone. West Indians encountering such barriers may harbour justifiable feelings of frustration.

LANGUAGES

The major language spoken varies with the island in question: English, French patois (a French-English dialect in areas colonized by the French), Spanish, Dutch, Portuguese, Hindi, and Creole (an English-African dialect, spoken in all the islands as a common language). In some situations in Canada, West Indians may speak in dialect or in their original language, especially if they have recently arrived, are among themselves, or under stress. However, English is fluently spoken by most and known by all.

RELIGION

Religion has always been central to West Indians. In the difficult times of slavery, and even now, religion has provided an avenue for optimism, hope for the future, and a means of social control to protect the society. The commonest religions are Roman Catholic, Protestant, Sikh, Muslim, and several others. Among Jamaicans, the Rastafarian religion is growing, and is becoming increasingly known to Canadians through its association with reggae music, the back-to-

Africa movement, and the Rastafarian belief in the divinity of the late Ethiopian Emperor Haile Selassie. In Canada, West Indians tend to attend church regularly and expect their children to cherish religious values.

PATTERNS OF MIGRATION

In the late 1950s and early 1960s, there was a heavy migration of West Indians to England for improved education and job opportunities. However, in 1962, the British government enacted a law discouraging the free entry of outsiders. As a result of stricter screening, fewer West Indians were able to enter England. At the same time, Canada relaxed its racial policies regarding immigration. As a result, during the late 1960s a great number of West Indians came to this country settling at first in the larger cities such as Toronto and Montreal, and later in western Canada. Male university students and female domestics were the commonest groups in the first wave to western Canada.

In the second wave of the early 1970s, West Indian migration to western Canada increased because of invitations from relatives and friends and better job opportunities. Many who came in this period were more financially secure, with established credentials, affluent families, and relatives who were already established in Canadian jobs. Many educated professionals from the West Indies were admitted to Canada by agreeing to accept work in deprived northern or rural areas in western Canada, and later settled in larger cities where West Indian cultural activities were accessible.

Of Canada's 250,000 Blacks and Caribbeans (constituting 10 per cent of Canada's overall population), 12 per cent or 30,000 now live in western Canada, 63 per cent or 157,500 in Ontario, 22 per cent or 55,000 in Quebec, and the remainder in the Maritimes. Most West Indians in western Canada live in the larger cities such as Winnipeg, Edmonton, Calgary, and Vancouver.

EXPERIENCE IN CANADA

Apart from being unaccustomed to the cold winters, West Indians in general have little difficulty adapting to life in Canada. This is perhaps partly because of the common British-influenced heritage and because of previous multicultural experience. West Indians tend to adapt rather than challenge the system.

Skin colour becomes especially important in western Canada because until recently there were relatively few visible minorities resident there. Most West Indians feel that they are accepted fairly well by Canadians, although they are fully aware that racism exists in both subtle and open forms: in employment, job promotion, education, and at social gatherings. However, few of them become preoccupied with this problem. At times, many may hesitate to confront racism actively. Group political action by West Indians in cases of known discrimination has only recently begun to develop. It has enjoyed the open support not only of the Black community, but also of many white Canadians who are concerned about human rights issues. Some white Canadian health professionals are initially uncomfortable about working with West Indian clients.

FAMILY STRUCTURE

Family structure in the West Indies usually varies with social class and ethno-cultural background. In many instances, however, the family consists of more than the nuclear unit living together. Married, grown-up children in the West Indies often live in or add another section to their parents' family home. Many cannot afford to buy land, since it is expensive. Sometimes a young couple will be expected to build their own dwelling before they can marry. These patterns may vary from island to island, and from one social class to another. Poorer families may form larger extended family groups for economic reasons. The extended family concept is practical and well accepted by most West Indians because of the companionship, support, and multiple sources of help which it offers.

Children born out of wedlock are common and no longer stigmatized, although instances have existed in the past where a family would go to great lengths to conceal such a child. In Jamaica, the term "illegitimate" is not used. A grandmother is grandmother to all her grandchildren, whether they come from a legal union or not. She may act as the link between the legitimized family and the additional members, and will not reject anyone.

A woman may remain single in the West Indies and have several children without being stigmatized. However, initial pregnancies among very young girls can occasion more disgrace and secrecy than later pregnancies. Although many couples remain faithful, longstanding extramarital liaisons are not uncommon. A man's wife may know about her husband's other partner, though she will not necessarily accept or be happy about the situation. Severe domestic quarrels may occur over these arrangements. Common law relationships are frequent and have always been well accepted.

Divorce has been rare in the past. Divorcing couples and their extended families may be strongly criticized and speculation may arise about possible weakness of character or shameful behaviour. Consequently, an unhappy marriage may be maintained while informal arrangements exist for extramarital relationships. Women exercising this option would be subject to much greater social disapproval than men, since "good behaviour" in general is differently defined for each sex. Westernization, however, is changing this pattern.

The extended family structure has some implications for Canadian health care. Health care workers in Canada may label the West Indian home as overcrowded if it contains many extended family members. In addition, a Canadian professional may expect that the eighteen-year-old to twenty-year-old person should be living independently, or paying rent to parents. In the West Indian family, however, family members may live at home as long as they wish. In Canada, the West Indian extended family, though not necessarily sharing housing, may include close friends and home town people with whom regular close contact is maintained over many years.

If severe family conflict arises such as might lead to divorce in other Canadian families, the West Indian family tends to remain together even at the cost of great individual unhappiness. In some cases, a blind eye may be turned to prevent family conflict and to enable the family to continue as a unit. Again, when embarrassing problems arise, the extended family resorts to privacy or secrecy to protect itself from gossip, disapproval, or group ridicule. It is important that the health care worker not make a larger issue of the situation than the family itself wishes to.

WEST INDIAN FAMILY STRUCTURE IN CANADA

The usual pattern of migration is that the husband, and possibly the wife, come to Canada first, leaving the children with their grandparents or aunts. Once the parents are settled in a job and home, they may send for the children. Often the children are not brought to Canada until they reach school age, in order to reduce the cost of child care. Even where children are born in Canada, they may be sent back home to grandparents or other extended family members for practical reasons, while the parents prepare for the child's return by establishing themselves in jobs and a home. The amount of money sent back for the child's support is comparatively small relative to child care costs in Canada.

When children do come to Canada, they may have difficulty adjusting to life with parents whom they scarcely know. They miss their extended family custodians and may have trouble making the transition to a mainly white society. For example, one eleven-year-old Jamaican child was reunited with her parents for the first time since she was five, and had difficulty relating to them. She joined a delinquent white peer group, which accepted her, and with whom she identified as being, like herself, outside mainstream school life. As a result of petty crimes, she was placed in a foster home, which she preferred to her parental home because the foster parents were white. Although it was actually the child who rejected her parents, the social worker viewed them as rejecting the child. Instead of working with the family to help maintain the West Indian extended family structure, the social worker violated this norm and placed the child outside the family.

Newly arrived West Indian children may feel that having a white friend is prestigious. They may defy their parents in order to achieve such friendships with equally lonely and alienated Canadian children. Antisocial behaviour may be typical of that group. Other parents in the West Indian community, faced for the first time with such behaviour, may view these children as impolite and poorly controlled by their parents, and may be concerned that their child will become antisocial too.

Two sources of alienation may trouble the newly arrived West Indian child: remoteness from natural parents who are strangers to them, and exclusion from the Canadian peer group. The health care worker can begin by seeking to understand the needs and concerns of the parents. The fact that they sent for the child is evidence of their sense of commitment and responsibility, and usually the parents genuinely want the best for the child.

Some problems can arise if the parents have already adopted some Canadian patterns to which the child is not accustomed. For example, the parents may offer only two full meals and a lunch snack, whereas the child may expect three full meals. As well, the child may be accustomed to the twenty-four hour support and presence of the extended family, whereas in Canada both parents may be at work when the child comes home from school. The child must occupy his or her own time, perhaps seeking companionship from children engaged in antisocial activities.

The health care worker may become involved in helping to solve such difficulties. Getting to know the family situation will greatly assist the worker in helping both parents and child to negotiate the mutual adjustments needed for the child to fit into the new life. Familiarity with the child's life in the West Indies will also be helpful. Although parents may assume that the child's experience in the

West Indies was positive, this may not have been the case. In some cases, children have had major drug or emotional problems in the West Indies, and become further stressed on relocation to Canada. Grandparents may not have informed the parents about such difficulties.

The health care worker can contribute to rebuilding family relationships in Canada, rather than to separating families. For example, one bright West Indian teenager heard the teacher say that he would "never make it" educationally, a comment which hurt and discouraged him. He withdrew, joined a group of rebellious students, and became a delinquent. Involvement with the juvenile justice system ensued, as did rejection by one parent, before the case was referred to a mental health worker, fortunately a West Indian person. The student was encouraged to enrol in a vocational program, where he began to experience success and show improved behaviour.

ROLES OF MEN AND WOMEN

Although no overall generalizations hold true for all families in the West Indies, there are some common themes. Women usually play a strong and decisive role within the household, while men assume more power over the affairs of the family in the outside world. In past generations, women's work was mainly within the home, where they assumed responsibility for all the cooking, cleaning, child care, and health care decisions. Mothers attended to the child's school progress and any problems which the teacher brought to her attention. The father took a back seat and the woman's decisions guided child care. Currently in Canada women may have some difficulty as they learn to take on more of the responsibilities outside the home, such as business arrangements, car maintenance, and so on. In turn, men may encounter problems in accepting their increased participation in domestic and child care tasks.

In the past, men mostly saw themselves as bread-winners, and as being responsible for heavier home jobs such as painting and fixing the house. With Westernization and greater economic demands more women work outside the home, so that some husbands share child care and other domestic duties such as cleaning or grocery shopping, though not always willingly. Professional families may instead decide to hire household help to perform these tasks.

Previously, it was mostly the men or single women who enrolled as students. Generally, a woman believed she had to choose between marriage or an advanced education, rather than combining the two. Currently, however, women may choose the latter option.

If funds for education are limited, the boy in the family will be given priority. In Indo-Caribbean families, it is expected that girls will marry and leave home, with the result that the son is more important to the future plans of the family. Consequently, Indo-Caribbean families may prefer the birth of a boy so that someone will be able to take over the family business and contribute to the family income.

There are different standards of conduct for each sex. Certain behaviours, acceptable for a boy, will be unacceptable in a girl. A good girl is one who has few if any boy-friends, doesn't stay out late, and is not talked about by others. A bad boy is so labelled, not for sexual conduct, but if he breaks the law, engages in destructive behaviour, or does poorly in school.

Social disapproval is a powerful means of controlling the behaviour of both sexes. Saving face is extremely important to the family, so that people may abstain from unacceptable conduct simply to avoid casting shame on the family. Fear of gossip in the social group will frequently restrain an individual from following his own wishes, a control not as strongly exercised in more individualistic Western societies. Rules for socially prescribed behaviour in both sexes are strongly maintained by the entire extended family group, not simply by the individual or his parents.

For example, if two teenagers "back home" are seen holding hands on the street, witnesses to this occurrence will inform the parents, and the children will be disciplined accordingly. As a result, children tend to become very secretive about their relationships. In Canada, West Indian parents may be much more tolerant of such behaviour. For adults, extramarital affairs may provoke gossip which in turn may lead to more discreet behaviour or even an end to the affair.

ROLE CHANGES IN CANADA

Migration to Canada has brought about some role changes in West Indian family life. In most families, both parents are now working, a situation not often true in the islands. As a result, the wife now has greater financial independence and is able to enjoy more freedom because she can afford child care. Thus, women are more liberated than they would have been had they not worked outside the home.

A West Indian couple may hold a joint bank account or may have individual accounts managed by each partner. Quite often it is the wife who takes care of routine bills and manages general household expenses including food and clothing. Some wives also manage their husband's business accounts, while others may have little contact with the family's overall financial affairs. As in Canadian marriages, mutual trust and individual ability and commitment are important factors in the degree of financial sharing. When wives are employed, joint financial arrangements are more common.

Role changes have occurred for grandparents too. In the past, where a husband and wife were both employed after settling in Canada, child care became necessary. One partner sometimes sent for a grandmother to look after the children, or sent a child back to the West Indies to be looked after by the grandparents.

Older West Indians coming to Canada under these arrangements often found life difficult. They sometimes felt that they were not given the respect or attention which they had received back home. Quite often they became lonely, isolated, and depressed, and complained about how much they missed their friends and the freedom of movement which they enjoyed in the West Indies. In Canada, this freedom was limited by the cold winters and transport problems. This situation often led to friction within the family. Some grandparents returned to the West Indies. Similarly, the children who were sent away to be raised in the West Indies, often encountered difficulties of adjustment on returning to the very different environment in Canada. Currently it is less common to bring grandparents to Canada or to send children back to them.

COURTSHIP AND MARRIAGE

In the past, and to a lesser extent currently, Indo-Caribbean families may arrange the marriages of their children far in advance. Now, some Indo-Caribbeans and most other groups follow a Western pattern, with teenagers dating under supervision and choosing their own partners. They meet in schools, homes, and parties. In Canada, teenagers of West Indian descent are usually allowed to mix freely with schoolmates in regular social gatherings. Newly immigrated West Indian parents may be unfamiliar with Canadian customs such as unsupervised teenage dances or younger children sleeping over at one another's home, and may be reluctant to allow it.

Some parents have difficulty when their young teenagers wish to stay out after 9:00 PM like their Canadian peers. Many parents living in the West Indies see such practices as irresponsible, and use stern physical punishment to control the child's activities. Types of punishment for both boys and girls may include a belt or switch.

EDUCATION

Education is very important to West Indian parents, most of whom want their children to advance as far as possible in school. Most parents regard a sound education as the best preparation for a good life, and a source of prestige for the family. It is especially prestigious to have offspring who work in the Civil Service, or study abroad. Older children may work and save so that younger children can be assisted to go away to study. Thereafter the older ones, having "paid their family dues," will be able to do likewise, often working their way through college.

In the past, during the first wave of immigration to Canada, only the rich could afford to send their children abroad to study. Thus the first West Indian students in Canada tended to be from upper, or upper-middle income levels. Lower-middle-class, or poor families with intelligent children, often made many sacrifices to obtain education. For the second wave of immigrants, however, more government educational scholarships became available to assist deserving students of all social levels to study away from home. Additionally, many now have relatives and friends already established in Canada with whom they can live, enabling them to study more easily.

Many current students are second or even third generation West Indian-Canadians, whose entire lives and those of their parents have been spent within the Canadian educational system. They will be less likely to be acquainted with "back home" health care practices than will recently arrived immigrants, and may be embarrassed if their parents or grandparents follow such practices.

A Canadian education increases the chances of West Indian people to find jobs appropriate to their education. Canadian credentials are more easily acknowledged, and a good understanding of the Canadian job situation is highly valued by potential employers. Immigrants coming with West Indian credentials, however, may encounter frustrating delays, both when seeking jobs, or when writing Canadian examinations to establish professional, technical, or trade equivalences. Subtle discrimination on the basis of colour is sometimes a barrier to career development, even where educational credentials are acceptable.

The recently arrived West Indian child, too, may be at some disadvantage within the Canadian school system. In Canada, it is expected that parents will take the initiative to keep abreast of school programs and children's progress by attending parent-teacher meetings. West Indian parents may hesitate to attend conferences with the teacher because of their respect for the teacher's authority. They may assume that the teacher will notify them of problems, as would be the case in the West Indies.

In the West Indies, school is regarded as an extension of the home, and the child is entrusted entirely into the teacher's hands. Teachers, who are expected to know what is best for the child's education, are more likely to keep in contact with parents over a child's progress. This is partly because of the individual initiative of the teachers, and partly because of the quick flow of information within the close community network. Either way, many school problems are quickly made known to the parents.

Sometimes, too, children's accents will cause teachers to underestimate West Indian pupils' abilities to learn. Even though English is the first language of most West Indians, the dialect may be difficult for some teachers to comprehend. The child may therefore seem backward to the teacher, and may be placed in a special classroom on the basis of a faulty assessment of academic ability. Instances arise where West Indian parents are unaware of (and therefore unable to rectify) the inappropriate placement of their children in classrooms for non-English speaking students or in vocational rather than academic courses.

DISCIPLINE

"Spare the rod and spoil the child" is a quotation often used by West Indian parents, who strongly believe in physical punishment. A child may be physically punished for misbehaviour or poor performance at school, in public, or at home. Strapping is commonly used both at home and school and is an accepted norm. West Indian parents in Canada may be aware that this is not so in Canada, but will still be inclined to discipline their children by this means. Although West Indian parents view it only as a way to improve the child's behaviour, Canadians may label it as child abuse and health authorities may charge parents accordingly. This results in much embarrassment and humiliation for the parent, who may then see the child as wrong in reporting them, and may even reject the child for doing so.

VALUES

Many of the values taught to West Indian children are imparted by parents, but are based on religion. These include respect for and obedience to authorities and elders. Cleanliness and grooming are very important to most families. Before children are presented in public, considerable attention will be paid to the cleanliness of the clothes and careful grooming of the hair. Children are expected to be seen and not heard. They are taught not to enter into conversation with adult visitors, and if they do so, may be sharply rebuked. Children are expected to listen to rather than challenge or argue with adults. Canadianized West Indian children, however, are much more inclined to challenge and interact with adults. This behaviour may upset parents and can lead to conflict between the generations.

For adults and children living in the West Indies, deep respect for the neighbours and authorities is central. Direct eye contact with elders or those in authority is not regarded as polite, but West Indian children and adults in Canada may expose themselves to criticism for being fearful, or even evasive, if they do not make eye contact at school or on the job. Children never address adults by their first names. They may be perceived by Canadians as unintelligent because of their lack of assertiveness with those in authority. Lack of confidence at school may lead to absenteeism. Children may have difficulty in establishing a place for themselves in the dominant culture, and this may lead to low self-esteem and lack of involvement at school.

Children who have recently arrived from the West Indies, acting out of customary good manners, may not speak up in class discussions or in conversations with professionals. Unless children are asked direct questions, and shown, through kind attention, that it is permissable to speak, they may remain silent. This may be evaluated by a teacher as passivity, ignorance, or stupidity. Intelligence may be further misjudged because standard psychological tests are culture-bound, and are designed mainly for the North American culture. Some questions or tasks may have little meaning for the first generation West Indian child.

This situation can easily lead the professional to make a false diagnosis or assessment of a child, which the parents in turn may not question out of respect for authority. When a health professional wishes to gain information about a child, the child should be encouraged to speak and be shown that his or her participation is acceptable and valued. Assessments made by other professionals should be accepted only tentatively until the professional concerned can validate them against approaches sensitive to West Indian norms for good manners. Otherwise, inaccurate assessments may lead to inappropriate health care and educational interventions.

NAMES

In the West Indies, it is common for the same person to be called by several different names by various people in his circle. A man is often called by his last name only, rather than by his first name or his title. Thus Prescott Brown becomes, to most people who know him, simply "Brown." He may also have a family name or "home name" such as "Junior," and this name may be used by all those close to him. In addition, he may have a nickname, derived from some abbreviation of his other names, his initials, or a personal characteristic. Thus a musician who plays lively music may be called "Pepper," and the Prime Minister of Trinidad-Tobago is known popularly by his initials, A.N.R.

If he is older, he may be referred to even by his closest friends of many years as "Mr. Brown." A child would never call an older person by the first name. Formality of address is also preferred in meeting strangers or professionals for the first time and West Indians generally expect to be addressed formally by professionals in return. Names are sequenced in the North American way, with the given names first, and the family name last.

PATTERNS OF COMMUNICATION

Hand movements are frequently lively, expressing aspects which go beyond the words spoken. Touching the arm, back, or shoulder is frequent in friendly social conversation. Little eye contact is used, to avoid seeming rude or intrusive. In conversation, people tend to glance briefly at a companion, and then look away rather than maintaining lengthier eye contact. With authority figures, the eyes may be averted during an entire conversation.

Expressions of physical affection are not a common part of West Indian family life or social life. In the past, couples rarely held hands or demonstrated affection in public because this behaviour was regarded as impolite, improper, and even shocking. Parents and children rarely hug or kiss one another openly, and generally do not verbalize direct statements of love, even in private.

Couples have physical contact mainly during sexual relationships. Sometimes, physical punishment by a jealous spouse is interpreted as a sign of deep caring. Affection between spouses is communicated mostly through actions such as going out shopping together, or socializing, or buying gifts. In Canada, West Indian patterns of communication may be similar to the traditional ones, or may resemble those of mainstream Canadians, depending upon each individual's degree of exposure to and acceptance of either type.

Envy and jealousy are common emotions in the West Indies. Envy over a person's new car might lead the carowner's friend to stop talking to him. Competition is keen over symbols of material success or wealth. "Keeping up with the Joneses" may produce much stress as people try to match or outdo each other. When people go to church they like to appear in new, fashionable clothing to show that they can afford expensive things. Much money is spent on appearances, even if strict economizing takes place behind the scenes on food and other less visible essentials.

West Indian language is rich in words to express feelings of jealousy about the ending of relationships. There may be several different terms depending on degree of painful lovesickness involved. For instance, in Trinidad, "tabanca" is the term for depression over losing a girl-friend. When a man is described as "getting horn," it means that his wife is being unfaithful to him. Acute loss of face results for the husband, who may be much ridiculed by others. Because of the personal pain involved when a relationship is failing, or an affair is discovered, secrecy is safeguarded as much as possible within the home. Either partner may eventually confide in a trusted friend or relative of the same sex, who may act as a go-between for the couple. However, they would not consult a professional for help, as they would not want their personal problems to be known or spread by outsiders. For this reason, they are unlikely to provide a health professional with adequate background information on marital and family problems, wife or child abuse, and so on. It is seen as a disgrace to wash the family's dirty linen in public.

Gossip is common. West Indian people regularly keep close contact with their friends and relatives by telephone. News and rumours travel fast and often become distorted along the way. When information is incomplete, gaps may be filled with guesswork, then passed along as truth, a pattern which is generally perpetuated in Canada.

West Indian people may use indirect methods of refusing invitations or requests. They may agree to attend or comply, and then fail to do so. This pattern may make it difficult for the health care worker who thinks that "yes" means agreement about the proposed plan of care when in fact, the person is only avoiding offensiveness. The Canadian health care worker may find it helpful to confirm an arrangement with a last-minute call, just to be sure. In such cases, polite greetings are in order first, prior to re-emphasizing the importance of the appointment.

It is common to engage in preliminary social chatter before getting down to the business at hand. Inquiries about the person's current activities, the well-being of his family, and other such topics are often used to sound out or break the ice with strangers. This use of social antennae enables one to gauge the receptiveness of the listener to the next communication. If the listener is unresponsive or hostile, the business may be left until another time when circumstances are more favourable. A health care worker can accomplish his or her task more effectively by engaging in such preliminary chatting. Mothers are likely to be pleased if their material possessions or the appearance and behaviour of their children are favourably commented upon. Small gifts for the children are also well received as a sign of goodwill.

CLOTHING

Generally, West Indians dress less casually than mainstream Canadians when they appear outside the home. Jeans are not commonly worn in the West Indies, whereas shirts, ties, and jackets are. Women may be more inclined to wear skirts or dresses than slacks. Some type of headgear is common for both sexes, and hairstyling is very important. As a group, most West Indians are very reluctant to be seen when not well groomed and well-dressed. Within the home, slippers may be worn. When in hospital, West Indian patients will much prefer to wear their own clothing rather than that provided by the hospital, since they do not feel comfortable or like to be seen wearing clothes that someone else has worn.

Other cultural groups, such as Indo-Caribbeans, may dress in saris and other traditional garments. West Indians may favour dressing well in public at the expense of important private needs, such as food, which can be cut down without public knowledge of hardship. In Canada, most West Indians, however, will dress like most other Canadians.

SHOPPING

Shopping may be either the wife's responsibility or a family outing. Wives usually shop for groceries and the children's clothing needs. They prefer expensive clothing and do not shop for bargains or second-hand items, partly out of considerations of status and partly to avoid social humiliation. Appliances, however, may be bought second-hand, and items which have a negotiable price in Canada, may indeed be bargained for. Otherwise, the marked price is paid without haggling or bargaining. Most avoid garage sales. Though the money is generally earned by the husband, it is often the woman who manages it, and she is free, within reasonable limits, to make the shopping decisions.

TIME

In the West Indies, the pace is slow. No one is in a rush and consequently people often arrive half an hour to one hour late for scheduled events. If a host wants people to arrive for eight o'clock, she or he might tell guests to come at seven. West Indians may therefore have difficulty in being punctual for medical appointments. However, they also hate to be kept waiting, and are impatient for things to start. If kept waiting too long, they may be inclined to leave and come back on another day.

West Indian businesses are not as time-bound as those in Canada. A shopkeeper opens his store when he gets there. If a customer finds a message that the shop will be open again in fifteen minutes, the period may, in fact, turn out to be an hour or two. These different time patterns may be difficult for Canadians to accept and may be interpreted as unreliability or irresponsibility.

Social events usually post a starting time which is several hours before the band will start playing or the main crowd is expected to arrive. Ticket-buying is left until the very last minute, since West Indian people do not like to schedule events too far ahead. Perhaps when the date of the event arrives it will not fit with their current inclinations. In both the West Indies and Canada, crowds for evening parties tend to arrive around 11:00 PM with parties lasting very late until 3:00 or 4:00 AM.

The West Indian emphasis is on people and process rather than time schedules and they may experience Canadian "efficiency" as impersonal and discourteous. Wherever feasible, the health care worker is likely to accomplish more by slowing down to match the pace of the patient.

RECREATION AND LEISURE

In Canada, many West Indian men continue to play their traditional cricket, soccer, and other sports. They have also brought with them some indoor board and card games such as rummy, dominoes, and all-fours. In addition, many have adopted Canadian sports such as bowling. Women in the West Indies traditionally spent their spare time visiting, or watching male sports, although in Canada subsequent generations of women may be more involved in community or professional activities.

Traditionally, it is the custom for West Indians to drop in unannounced at any time to visit relatives, friends, and neighbours. In Canada, some prefer a prior call and a few others insist upon being notified and do not receive unannounced visitors. Community health care workers who call first are more likely to be received by the latter group.

A great number of West Indians spend their leisure time in church and organizational activities. Generally, they are a very friendly people who greatly enjoy socializing, especially on weekends, whether it be at home or at social gatherings held by the various West Indian organizations in Canada.

WEST INDIES HEALTH SYSTEM

In most of the West Indian islands basic medical care is paid for by the government. However, sometimes services offered by clinic and hospital are slow and take place in poorly equipped, poorly staffed, or inconveniently located facilities. In the main, however, most urban medical facilities are operated by well-trained West Indian doctors, nurses, and technicians who receive their education in England, the United States, and Canada, or from the University of the West Indies in Jamaica or Trinidad.

Minor illnesses such as colds, flu, earaches, headaches, toothaches, and asthma are treated at home because of the patient's preference, cost, proximity of doctor or hospital, or the infrequency of scheduled clinics in rural areas. Major physical illnesses such as heart attacks, cancer, diabetes, and persistent pains are treated in hospitals, clinics, or by private doctors. Those who can afford to will usually be treated by a private doctor or in a private hospital.

Although, in the past, financial means were a major determinant of the type of care chosen, this picture has changed. Economic barriers in the West Indies have been somewhat lowered by improved wages, and by the provision of a better quantity and quality of free health care services. Money only partly influences the West Indian's choice of traditional or non-traditional health care.

FOLK MEDICINE AND WESTERN MEDICINE

Many West Indians today still use herbal or "bush" medicine as a cure for their illnesses. In the past, it was used especially by those people living in rural areas, those from a lower socio-economic group who could not afford a doctor, and those who did not have immediate access to clinics or hospitals. However, there are still many West Indians both at home and in Canada who, regardless of their education or socio-economic background, use some combination of traditional and Western medicine. Herbal remedies often prove highly effective. In Canada, however, use of herbal medicine may be limited by unavailability of the traditional herbal ingredients.

Treatment of illness often rests upon religious beliefs. Belief in spirit possession is common to certain folk religions in the West Indies. In some cases of illness those who have a strong belief in the supernatural will call upon the assistance of the clergy, or resort to the magic of the obeah man. Obeah is a system of belief and practice involving manipulation of evil spirits.

Many West Indians believe in the devil as a real and powerful force who is responsible for the occurrence of unusual behaviour or harmful acts. When the cause of illness or misfortune is unknown, for example in mental illness, cancer, or oedema of the legs, some people are inclined to think that an evil supernatural power is at work. A person with schizophrenic hallucinations may be seen as having a devil in him.

As a natural outcome of this belief, some families will seek help from a person who can make religious or supernatural interventions. For example, a girl of sixteen who believed that the radio was speaking to her as the voice of God, began talking back to the radio. Her parents were worried and helpless, and neighbours came around in curious groups to stare. Thinking she was possessed by the devil, her family responded by calling the priest to pray for the girl. Eventually, however, she was taken to a doctor and hospitalized.

In the West Indies the rich, the middle class, and those who live in cities where adequate health services are available are more likely to seek biomedical care. Medical intervention would also be sought by those for whom "bush" medicine or other folk remedies have not cured persistent pains or serious illnesses. For example, a woman diagnosed with breast cancer could not afford to pay for the medication prescribed by a physician. She then turned to an obeah man, in the belief that her cancer was caused by a brassière which she had been given by another woman and through which a spell had been passed. Some West Indians, however, fully trust modern health care and use doctors and hospitals in the same way as Canadians do.

The countries of the English-speaking Caribbean have made considerable progress in developing better health care policies and services (Carr 1985). The degree to which modern medicine is used in the islands often depends upon its availability, cost, and patient preference. Urban areas are much better served than rural areas. Some islands today have well-equipped and well-staffed hospitals, travelling clinics, and private physicians while others may lack some of these resources. The degree to which new immigrants use Western medicine will depend upon their previous experiences and beliefs at home in the islands.

Public health care and hospital care in the West Indies are free. Diagnosis and treatment are mostly provided in scheduled outpatient clinics, which may be set up at infrequent intervals in outlying areas. Many doctors view private practice rather than hospitals or clinics as their service priority. People who wish to consult a private physician must have financial means, since private consultation can be very costly. Wealthier people may prefer to have their own private physician as a matter of pride. If a doctor is reputed to be good in certain areas, such as cancer, people will line up to see him. West Indians tend to put much faith in the individual professional.

Because hospitals are viewed as places to die, many West Indians try to avoid them unless they are seriously ill, especially if the hospitals near them are overcrowded, unhygienic, or poorly maintained. However, some large city hospitals are clean and efficient and are the preferred setting for childbirth and the treatment of serious conditions.

In rural areas, trained midwives assist with all or most of the home births. Usually, a midwife delivers the baby at the homes of poorer families; she stays two or three days and is assisted by family members. The husband, although he stays close by, will not be present in the delivery room. Middle- or upper-income families may choose to give birth in hospitals or private nursing homes, whereas poorer families only go to hospital if there are complications during labour. In Canada, West Indians' use of hospitals varies depending on past experience in the West Indies.

In the West Indies, most professionals are regarded with very deep respect and deference. Since health professionals are so highly respected, patients may regard the medical visit itself as the cure rather than any health care action which they themselves may take. For example, if medication has been prescribed, the patient may discontinue using it upon only slight improvement, regarding his visit to the doctor as the curative factor. This occurs in Canada as well. Antibiotics or other courses of medication may be taken only until the patient feels better, rather than for the length of time specified. As well, many people experience considerable embarrassment about revealing their bodies to health care professionals. For example, one West Indian immigrant in northern Manitoba complained only of severe pain in the left side of her abdomen, when a prolapsed uterus was fully visible externally. She was unable to mention this symptom directly.

Despite the availability of medical care in Canada, many first generation West Indians in Canada may not seek regular check-ups, tending to treat minor illnesses at home before consulting a doctor. Some need considerable encouragement in making timely use of the medical system.

DISEASES

Some of the diseases more common to the West Indies than Canada are poor teeth, tropical skin diseases, and children's worms, rickets, and hepatitis. Previously common diseases such as tuberculosis, poliomyelitis, diphtheria, and measles are now very rare. As elsewhere, AIDS now occurs in the West Indies and is a public concern. Stigma is attached to diseases which once had a fatal prognosis, such as tuberculosis, since people fear that the infected person will contaminate others. Mental illness is also stigmatized because of the belief that the person may be possessed by the devil.

MENTAL ILLNESS

If a man is depressed and withdrawn in the West Indies, he is not generally viewed as being sick, and therefore is not likely to seek psychiatric help. Instead, he will be described by family and friends as "havin' worries" or "studyin' [thinking] too much." With the family's support, and the solace and companionship of the local "rum shop," he very often comes out of the depressive period. The rum shop sells drinks by the bottle or glass, and is the place where men congregate to talk with friends. After a few drinks, problems may be discussed more uninhibitedly and gossip is not a common consequence of personal disclosures. For most West Indians, male or female, depression will not be displayed openly except to a good friend who will provide support through the bad period. Frequently both physical and psychological pain will be hidden under a show of strength, since revelation of problems in general may be viewed as weakness. The person displaying schizophrenic hallucinations or delusions will be thought of as being possessed by the devil and taken to a clergyman or obeah man for help.

Psychiatric help is not as readily available in the West Indies as in Canada. Since not every island has a mental institution, admission may involve moving far from home, perhaps to another island. Generally, the only people who are admitted to a mental institution are those who constitute a great danger to themselves or others. Since there is a powerful stigma attached to mental illness, few families want others to know that they have a mentally ill member. Consequently, due to both distance and stigma, families are likely to keep mentally ill persons at home as long as possible. If they have to be institutionalized, families are unlikely to visit them.

Hospital stays tend to be long. Treatment usually includes medication and physical restraint, but not psychological treatment such as individual, group, family, or occupational therapy.

Vocational rehabilitation programs are beginning to help the patient re-enter the community. However ex-psychiatric patients have difficulty in regaining community acceptance. Consequently, fear of stigma may prevent West Indian immigrants in Canada from seeking psychiatric treatment. This helps to explain their apparently low general usage of Canada's mental health system.

Because of current economic and social changes in the West Indies, stress is gaining recognition as a problem. West Indians now may complain about stress or "bein' under a lot of pressure." Symptoms of stress might include irritability, quarrelling, increased drinking, or being difficult. Family tension may increase, with verbal or at times physical abusiveness to spouse and children. Causes of stress may include job loss, illness, family conflict, poor school performance by children, financial problems, homesickness in a new country, or a sense of not getting ahead in life.

SUICIDE

In the West Indian islands, the rate of suicide, though not high generally, is commonest where individuals feel that they have failed or lost face in the social group. This is especially true of the Indo-Caribbean population. Methods of suicide are potent, and usually successful. Hanging, and the drinking of poisonous weed-killer ("Indian Tonic") are two of the commonest methods of suicide in the Indo-Caribbean groups. A major precipitant of female suicide is a failed romance. Suicide is often blamed on the family. Family and friends may know the real cause, but are likely to keep both the fact of the suicide and its cause a secret from the community at large. They may fabricate plausible accounts to tell others.

Among West Indians in western Canada, suicide appears to be

very rare. Possible reasons for this may include greater independence in making choices, and less pressure from the extended family in major life decisions. Perhaps in Canada, failure to accomplish career, marriage, and educational goals is less common, or independent coping skills are better developed.

SELF-PRESCRIPTION AND TRADITIONAL HEALING IN CANADA

Although most West Indians in western Canada readily use Canadian medicine for serious, acute, or chronic illnesses, they may first try their traditional remedies for minor complaints, before going to a doctor. It is important for the health professional to inquire from the patient what he has already tried, over what length of time, and whether or not it has been effective. Some people may not admit to using their own remedies for fear of being branded as backward, not only by doctors but also by fellow West Indians. Traditional remedies may not be readily available in Canada, and therefore will be replaced by easily obtainable over-the-counter remedies, or in more serious instances, by prescribed medications.

SLEEPING PATTERNS

In the West Indies, some of the homes of very large families may have only one or two bedrooms. Various arrangements will be used to accommodate sleeping members. In some cases, all males may sleep in one room and all females in the other, or the smaller children may sleep with their parents. In Canada, homes tend to be more spacious, and families smaller in size. In the West Indies, many people go to bed very early, about 9:00 PM, especially in the rural areas where work must start very early to beat the heat of the afternoon. In Canada, bedtimes may be later because of different working hours, longer daylight, and the availability of evening shopping and entertainment.

BATHING AND ELIMINATION

Often in the West Indies, bathing and elimination patterns depend upon the availability of a plentiful water supply. In the dry season, water is sometimes rationed so that people do not use indoor toilets and may take fewer baths. Overall, it is common for West Indians to shower twice a day, in the morning and the evening. Some rural homes have outdoor, non-flush toilets. Purges are commonly used for constipation.

In Canada, West Indians' bathing and elimination patterns resemble those of other Canadians. It may be necessary to provide explanations and privacy if a urine or stool sample is to be collected, since embarrassment discourages this procedure, as it does bathing in hospital. A patient may prefer to be bathed by a close relative rather than by a nurse. Women's bodies in particular are regarded as very private.

FOOD PATTERNS

The traditional West Indian diet tends to be high in starches, and features foods such as roti (flat bread wrapped around a curried meat and potato stew mixture), plantain (a starchy banana-type fruit used as a vegetable), peas and rice (an economical mixture providing a complete protein combination), breadfruit, cassava root, and so on. Meat dishes include highly seasoned curries made from chicken, beef, and goat. Favourite vegetables include green, spinach-like calaloo which is cooked with small amounts of water, fat, and salt pork. Salt fish is common as a less expensive dish, and seasoned, fresh fried fish is also a favourite. Fruits such as mangoes and papayas are more readily available in the West Indies than in Canada. Oranges and home-made ice cream are also often enjoyed as desserts. It is possible that the high starch and sugar diet may contribute to the high incidence of diabetes in the West Indies.

In the West Indies, three heavy meals a day are common. A typical West Indian breakfast consists of unfilled roti bread, four to six slices of toast, bacon, eggs, and coffee. Dinner, the midday meal, may include rice and stew, soup, and dumplings. Again at supper, a meat dish is often served. This pattern is changing in Canada, but island visitors to homes in Canada may be unhappy if not served the customary three heavy meals.

Members of other West Indian cultural groups, such as Indo-Caribbeans or Chinese, follow their own food patterns both in the West Indies and in somewhat changing degree in Canada. Hindus do not eat beef, since the cow is regarded as sacred. Older Hindus may eat with the right hand rather than with utensils. Muslims do not eat pork. Some religious groups are vegetarian and will eat eggs and fish but not meat. Fasting is practised by Muslims. Health care interventions in Canada such as surgery or a barium meal may need to be timed to avoid traditional fasting periods.

The Sunday meal is the family's weekly feast in the Caribbean. A three-course meal with all the trimmings is served at midday. Even if a family cannot afford meat any other day of the week, it will be served, along with the best obtainable fresh vegetables from the market, on Sunday.

Holiday celebrations include the killing of a goat or pig at Christmas, and preparation of coconut cake, rum cake, punchicreme (a spiced sweet rum and milk drink), mauby (a bitter tasting drink made from the bark of a tree), ginger beer, sorrel (made from a sweetened infusion of red leaves), rum punch, and spicy meat pastries called patties or pasties. At Easter, Christians eat fish instead of meat.

Certain foods are either avoided as taboo or prescribed. For example, it is believed that one should not eat bananas at night, since they are regarded as hard to digest. Cold foods are not eaten at night either, since they might upset the stomach. Pregnant women "eat for two," while children are given whatever the adults eat. Ill people are often fed soups made of beef or chicken.

Generally, the older generation of West Indians in Canada follows traditional food patterns as much as possible within limitations of supply and cooking time. Even West Indian wives who work outside the home will cook traditional dishes every weekend. However, their children may choose foods similar to those eaten by Canadian young people, such as hamburgers and French fries, and may object to traditional dishes.

In Canada, many West Indians find hospital food bland and tasteless, and prefer relatives to bring in more highly seasoned foods. These may be detrimental to the patient's condition since the relatives do not understand the principles of the therapeutic diet. For example, one man with ascites (fluid retention in the abdomen) was on a low salt diet which he disliked and which his relatives supplemented with well salted, highly seasoned foods. The patient ate these foods in secret, unknown to nurses. For other patients, a return to seasoned foods after surgery may cause abdominal discomfort. Patients should therefore be advised as to the foods most appropriate to recuperation and have the reasons for these choices and their importance carefully explained.

ALCOHOL

Liquor laws in the West Indies are not restrictive. Liquor is readily available in grocery shops and in the local rum shops, which also serve as places for men to gather and socialize over a glass or bottle of rum. It is, however, a disgrace for women to drink or smoke in public. People may drink on the street, or while driving cars, so that alcohol abuse is a significant problem. However, the resulting fatalities have not led to campaigns to change the liquor laws. Alcohol is also used hospitably on social occasions, such as weddings, wakes, and carnival celebrations.

In Canada, West Indian women tend to drink only a small amount of alcohol, whereas men use larger quantities. Alcoholism, though common among West Indians, is not seen as a disease needing treatment unless there are physical problems. Alcohol consumption can create abuse in the family, but will still not be labelled as a drinking problem. With Canada's stricter liquor and driving laws, an impaired person may be forced to undergo treatment in order to retain his driving license. As a result there are currently more West Indians in alcohol treatment programs than there were in previous years.

ILLEGAL DRUGS

Although most young West Indians growing up in their home countries have been exposed to illegal drugs, they may or may not use them here. Those raised in western Canada are often conservative in terms of illegal drug use.

DENTAL PRACTICES

In the West Indies, most people use commercial toothbrushes if they can afford them; if not they may use an hibiscus stick as a substitute. Salt may be used in place of toothpaste, and charcoal is sometimes used for making the teeth white. In Canada, West Indian dental practices are likely to resemble those of mainstream Canadians.

CHILDBIRTH

In the West Indies, childbirth usually occurs at home, in a private nursing home, or in the hospital, depending upon cost, availability of services, and the family's preference. A midwife generally delivers the baby, and the majority of mothers breast-feed. The mother rests for a few days, though not in seclusion, and she enjoys showing off the new baby to visiting friends and relatives. Postpartum depression is rare. In Canada, childbirth is likely to occur in hospital.

CARE OF THE AGED

In the West Indies, elderly people are cared for in the home, except for the very rich who may place the elder in a private nursing home. Usually, a daughter or daughter-in-law cares for the parents, but if there are no children, a brother or sister will do so. Sometimes if family members are unavailable a close female neighbour or friend may assume such care.

Old persons who cannot be managed at home may go to a hospital for the aged but this is not a popular option. These hospitals have poorhouse connotations, because most occupants are vagrants or without family. It is shameful for families not to treat their aged members well since old people are much respected and good treatment is considered their due.

Caring for aged West Indians is not yet a public problem in Canada. Although ailing parents may be brought to Canada to receive good medical care, most are younger and many plan to return to the West Indies when they retire. However, elderly West Indians now living in Canada sometimes experience loneliness as they miss the social ties with friends in the homeland. Religious worship, a source of support for many West Indians, may not be available in familiar form.

As Western influences increase, the grandparents' place in the hierarchy is gradually being eroded. Grandparents visiting Canada may want to take over direction of childcare just as they would at home, but parents here may be unco-operative, fearing a loss of their Canadian parental identity. One grandmother objected to a child's "disrespectful" speech and thought that the mother should take action. When she did nothing, the grandmother took punitive action herself. This event caused enough conflict for the mother to ask the grandmother to leave.

Because of the decline in their traditional role, grandparents lose their sense of identity and position, and may become unhappy enough to return to the West Indies. Their age and experience may no longer be respected in Canada. First generation West Indian Canadians are then caught between two worlds. They may wish to care for ageing parents but struggle to do so in ways which conform with their more independent lives in Canada. If the parent returns to the West Indies, citing mistreatment, those back home will blame the Canadian member for failing in an important social duty.

DEATH AND DYING

In the West Indies, most people die at home, using hospitals only as a last resort. Many West Indians are afraid of death, believing that the wandering spirit of the dead person may cause trouble to others.

Spirits of people who die a natural death, such as from old age, are less feared than those of people who die untimely deaths, by accident or violence. If the normal life span is regarded as fifty-five years, the soul of a person who dies unnaturally at forty-five may be thought of as hovering near the earth for the remaining ten years.

It is often thought that a restless soul can take living people into the next world. People will therefore be afraid to approach the body of a person who dies unnaturally or prematurely. They will also hurry past a spot on the road where a fatal accident has occurred. The spirit of a young child who dies before being christened is called a "dwen," and is thought to stay for an indefinite time on earth, where it wanders in the bushes and leads people astray.

West Indians believe that if a shooting star appears to fall on someone's house, a person in that family will die. The sound of a howling dog or a hooting owl is also thought to foretell death. Dreams are regarded as very significant, and are taken seriously. A person born with a "veil" over the face is regarded as having the ability to see or sense evil spirits which are invisible to others.

Indo-Caribbeans believe in reincarnation. If people behave and live well in this life, they will be born back into a good life the next time. Therefore, death of a good person is not regarded as very upsetting. Suffering, however, may be seen as divine retribution for errors or sins in past lives.

The amount of grief displayed at the death may be related to the degree of concern that the remaining members have for the soul of the dead. Those persons who did not lead a good life or who died an untimely death give rise to greater worry and grief. A death from cancer may also be regarded as untimely. The body will be prayed over for a full day in a ceremony called "bhagwat," in order to purify the soul and alleviate the distress of the dead person. Tears are less common in grieving in the West Indies than in some other Western countries.

Both Indo-Caribbean and Afro-Caribbean families hold wakes on the night of the death and many go on continuously night and day until the body is buried or cremated. These are gatherings in which kin, neighbours, and even strangers sing hymns, pray, eat specially prepared food, drink, play cards, and talk. The atmosphere may be quite happy. Wakes seem to be occasions for the community to lend moral support to the grieving family, and to affirm the life of the group, even though a member is dead.

In the West Indies people often have a further wake on the ninth day after death, known as "Nine Nights." In some islands it is also the custom to wash all the clothes of the dead person, as if to purify them. People then get together again to pray and sing, have coffee, biscuits, and liquor. Gambling is a feature of these gatherings and often travelling gamblers join whatever wake is currently in progress.

In Canada, many of these practices are modified or dropped. The health care worker, however, should be aware that expressions of grief may not be as overt as for other groups, and that allowance should be made for an influx of visitors to view the dead person. Usually, a dying elder will call someone significant in the family to hear a final message such as instructions about caring for certain members in the future.

There are no particular customs for treating the body after death. Most West Indians prefer not to have a post mortem since once death has happened they are not interested in knowing the technical details about its cause. If a post mortem is to be performed, its necessity should be clearly explained to the family.

In Canada, because West Indian deaths are rare and are generally from unexpected, accidental causes, families may be totally unprepared to deal with them. Canadian funeral arrangements may be confusing and unfamiliar to first generation immigrants. Families may need information about the inevitable formalities that follow deaths, such as dealing with the bank, insurance, and funeral arrangements.

DELIVERING CULTURALLY SENSITIVE HEALTH CARE

There are several key points that health professionals may find useful in working with West Indians in Canada. First, individual use of the Canadian health system will be affected by degree of belief in traditional bush or herbal medicine, and by prior experience of and faith in Western medicine.

Many West Indians have great respect for professionals and find it difficult to interact openly with them. Further, there is considerable insistence on confidentiality. West Indians may fear loss of face in their social group if their health problem is known and may withhold important information. This may be due to embarrassment, uncertainty about the professionals' confidentiality, or because they do not wish to impart more than they think is strictly relevant.

Lack of trust may lead the person to tell only part of the truth. Unless the professional is able to explain the relevance and importance of a thorough assessment and assure the person of confidentiality, incomplete data is more likely to be given. Invasion of privacy is a central concern for West Indian people, and may block both the free flow of information, and undressing the body. The visit to the doctor may be kept secret even from the patient's spouse. Medical check-ups are not usually sought because doctors are associated with serious diseases while hospitals are only thought appropriate to life-threatening illness.

Most West Indians, especially men, do not like going to doctors or hospitals unless it is a matter of life and death. Men, in particular, view requests for help as an admission of weakness. In emergency departments where busy nurses collect data to assess the potential severity of the problem, the information gathered will at times be insufficient or incorrect. This may be due to communication barriers such as the patient's accent or his ignorance of the terminology used for his ailments. He may also be reluctant to give information which he feels has nothing to do with his present complaints. As a result he may withhold additional details thus inviting incorrect investigation, diagnosis, or treatment.

It is important for the health professional, when encountering difficulties in understanding, to ask the person to speak more slowly or to point to the affected area of the body. It will also be helpful if the person taking a medical or social history explains the purpose of routine questions which the patient may not easily relate to his condition.

The client who has recently arrived from the West Indies may not be familiar with the roles and functions of various health care personnel in Canada. Explanations of the resources available to him or her may be helpful. Having chosen a physician, the West Indian client may be reluctant to change to another, since establishing trust involves surmounting considerable initial barriers and the person may not wish to start all over again. Immigrants will not usually choose a West Indian physician for fear that their personal information will get back to the community or that they will have to face the professional at the next social event.

Many people of West Indian origin in Canada are fully cognizant of medical procedures and well able to communicate their health problems to professionals. The task of the health care professional is to learn about individual West Indians in order to gauge how applicable the information presented in this chapter is to each case.

One further caution. Although the term "West Indian" implies one culture, each island is distinctly different from the others. Terminology and approaches to various health problems may differ considerably within and between islands.

FURTHER READING

Carr, P.R. "Health Systems Development in the English-speaking Caribbean: Towards the 21st Century," *Bulletin of the Pan American Health Organization*, Vol. 19, No. 4 (1985):368–83

"Communicable Diseases in the Caribbean," *Bulletin of the Pan American Health Organization*, Vol. 19, No. 4 (1985):396–99

Fisher, Lawrence. *Colonial Madness: Mental Health in the Barbadian Social Order*. New Brunswick, NJ: Rutgers University Press, 1985

Mitchell, M.F. "Popular Medical Concepts in Jamaica and Their Impact on Drug Use," *The Western Journal of Medicine*, Vol. 139, No. 6 (1983):37–43

Parmar, M.D. "Family Care and Ethnic Minorities," *Journal of Clinical Nursing*, Vol. 2, No. 36 (1985):1068–71

Pyme-Timothy, H. "Cultural Integration and the Use of Trinidad Creole," *Journal of Caribbean Studies*, Vol. 5, No. 4 (1986):7–15

CONTRIBUTORS

Edris Bridgewater
Selwyn Burt
Ann Carlyle
Nick Cumberbatch
Elizabeth Dickson
Vincent D'Oyley (UBC)
Seech Gadjadarsingh
Noga Gayle

Joan Hanuman
Dorian Ince
Sybil Joseph
Barbara Lashley
Keith Mondesir
Sandy Persaud
Yvonne Robinson
Barbara Thompson

CHAPTER TEN

Conclusion: Delivering Culturally Sensitive Health Care

Joan M. Anderson, Nancy Waxler-Morrison, Elizabeth Richardson, Carol Herbert, and Maureen Murphy

The ethnic composition of western Canada has become increasingly diverse over the past decades, with many immigrants and refugees coming from countries in South and Southeast Asia, Central America, and the Caribbean. The health beliefs and practices of the newcomers often differ markedly not only from the mainstream population, but also from the health professionals who provide care. This book has presented some basic facts about some immigrant groups in western Canada. A central argument throughout is that cultural categories confer specific meanings on the experience of illness. The authors have also shown that culture and ethnicity are not the only factors that influence health beliefs and practices. The socio-economic circumstances of people's lives, their political experiences in their home countries, and the way health care services in Canada are organized all play a major part in determining newcomers' experiences, their help-seeking behaviours, and how they manage health and illness.

Health professionals caring for patients from a particular ethnic group will want to consult the appropriate chapter. However, as we reviewed the chapters it became apparent that there are recurrent issues among the ethnic groups discussed.

This chapter therefore discusses the common themes throughout the chapters that shed light on the lives of the majority of immigrants and refugees to western Canada, and discusses practical guidelines for the delivery of health care services to these groups.

COMMON THEMES

Understanding Intraethnic Diversity and Avoiding Ethnic Stereotypes

A central point stressed throughout the book is that while there are usually shared beliefs, values, and experiences among people from a given ethnic group, quite often there is also widespread intra-ethnic diversity. Factors such as social class, religion, level of education, and area of origin in the home country (rural or urban) make for major differences within immigrant groups. These factors influence patients' beliefs about health and illness, their help-seeking behaviour, their expectations of health professionals, and their practices regarding health and illness. In Chapter 7 on South Asians, for example, it was noted that people come not only from a variety of regions with different languages and dialects, but also from several distinct religious groups. The Chinese living in western Canada, as Chapter 4 indicates, also come from different regions and countries with different languages and dialects, and great variation in experience.

Furthermore, in some countries a small urban élite enjoys a high standard of living, whereas a large number of people from both urban and rural areas live at subsistence level. These variations make for major differences in health beliefs and practices. For example, notions about the use of biomedicine, the place of preventative health care, and the concept of rehabilitation may vary among people from the same ethnic group. Whereas members of the upper classes are usually familiar with, and have access to, the latest in medical technology from the West and can afford excellent care on a par with European and North American standards, this is not the case with the urban poor and rural populations.

A point emphasized by the authors is the need to avoid ethnic stereotyping as ethnic factors operate in varying degrees in the lives of people with whom health professionals will come into contact. That is, some people closely follow the traditional practices of the home country, while others may not believe in such traditions. Among others, components of the traditional culture are built into an otherwise "modern" lifestyle. Conversely, persons who may appear "traditional" may be familiar with many aspects of the Western way of life. For example, it should not be assumed that if a woman wears a sari she will use traditional health care practices or is unfamiliar with English. In fact, health professionals often assume quite incorrectly that if persons are dressed differently they will not understand English and will be "different." Neither should it be assumed that a patient who is dressed in Western clothes and speaks fluent English will necessarily understand the Canadian way of doing things. Obtaining the details of the person's story is the only way to find out what he or she believes or expects.

Problems of Resettlement in a New Country

Although ethnic particularities cannot be denied, there are shared experiences among people who settle in a new country. These experiences, embedded within the social and economic conditions of people's lives in Canada, play a significant part in the experience of health and illness.

As we have pointed out, people come from different backgrounds in their countries of origin. Some were professionals and enjoyed a certain prestige and a reasonable standard of living. Migration to Canada was seen as a way to achieve an even higher standard of living and to secure a good future for their children. Others did not have the option to migrate. Many, because of political strife in their homelands, fled their countries in search of refuge here. And many saw Canada as the "promised land" where they could start over and make a better life for themselves and their children.

However, many have been disappointed by the realities of life in Canada. Upon their arrival here, many professional people have had to take menial jobs to make a living. Lacking fluency in English and Canadian qualifications, they cannot practise their professions; to survive, they have to take whatever jobs they can find. Although they came to Canada for a better life, their experience is one of downward socio-economic mobility.

Some immigrants are from the lower socio-economic groups in their countries of origin, and were therefore not able to obtain a high level of education. They may have difficulty learning English even after several years domicile in Canada, particularly if they could not read or write their own home language. With access only to low paying jobs, many are faced with a life of poverty and despair.

Social and economic factors then, and not ethno-cultural ones, may contribute to a person's depression and/or psychosomatic illnesses. This means that health professionals have to be constantly aware of the total context of people's lives, and the hardships that come from the process of uprooting and resettlement. Coping with a new language and with major changes in lifestyle, trying to find and keep a job, and dealing with government bureaucracies are some of the major stresses in the lives of immigrants and refugees. For visible, dark-skinned, non-English speaking minority groups, the problem of racism in neighbourhoods, schools, workplace, and health care institutions may be real. The stresses that a newcomer to Canada faces are often heightened when there is an illness, and especially when there are few sources of support.

Furthermore, many immigrants working in low paid, menial jobs do not have the benefits other Canadians take for granted, such as sick time and time off work to see a doctor. Many work in non-unionized jobs and get paid for the hours they are actually on the job. These factors add to the stresses of illness. From their reports, economic factors are usually paramount in the lives of many immigrants, and influence illness management and help-seeking. For example, failure to keep clinical appointments or to buy medicines could be the result of economic rather than ethno-cultural factors.

Health professionals need to keep in mind that people who migrated to Canada voluntarily bring a different set of experiences from refugees who were compelled to leave their countries out of concern for their personal safety. Many refugees left behind their possessions and loved ones, often not knowing if their relatives were dead or alive. Many want to go back "sometime" in the hope that they will find and be reunited with their loved ones.

A large number of refugees have been the victims of torture. Gleave and Manes, in writing about Central Americans in Chapter 3, note that physicians examining refugee claimants frequently find evidence of violence and torture. The pain of the refugee experience goes far beyond these physical wounds. They point out that children are haunted by nightmares of murders they have witnessed, adults are plagued by sleeplessness, and families mourn for those killed, imprisoned, or who have "disappeared." Compassion and sensitivity are needed by health professionals in dealing with people who have not only experienced immense suffering in their home country, but who may also be disappointed with their lives in Canada. Many have to settle for menial jobs and low pay. Even when incomes are meagre there are still obligations to be met; many must support relatives in the home country. Disenchanted with their own lives, and seeing no way to improve their situations, they begin to place hope in their children, only to discover that the children have become "too Canadianized."

The difficulties experienced by refugees may not easily be shared with others outside the immediate family. Language barriers, the perceived "coolness" of Canadian neighbours, a feeling of marginality in Canadian society, and unfamiliarity with the way of life here, all add to the sense of isolation. While immigrants may experience Canadian society in similar ways, the refugee may find life more difficult, as "returning home" is usually not an option.

Gender-Related Issues and Family Adjustment

The issues surrounding gender and family life are central to this book and are relevant to the delivery of health care services. One issue pertains to the role of women in other societies and the changes that occur on migration to Canada. In some groups the man is traditionally the bread-winner, while the woman takes care of the home. Out of economic necessity, however, many immigrant women must find employment outside the home. The family as a unit benefits economically from the woman's income, and some women find that they gain the respect of their husbands by making a financial contribution to the family. Nevertheless, role changes within the family sometimes lead to family conflict. As women become more aware of their rights in Western society, and as they become more independent, the man may grow to resent the Westernization of his wife. Furthermore, a man may feel that he has lost status within the family if he is unable to fulfil the role of being the bread-winner. In other words, he may lose face.

Both men and women go through a process of readjustment in order to cope with their lives in Canada. Women may find this process especially difficult when their own families have not immigrated to Canada, and when they are part of their husbands' households. They may have few sources of support in their community. Many women fear that airing family problems outside the home will provoke gossip in the community, and may eventually get back to the family. So, even though women may be part of a large extended family, they may still feel socially isolated as they have no one to turn to for help with personal problems.

Divorce is not usually an acceptable option for women from many groups, as women are brought up to believe that keeping a marriage together is their responsibility. Furthermore, divorce and separation stigmatize a woman and may lead to rejection by her ethnic community. She may therefore choose to remain with her husband even though the marriage is unsatisfactory, since facing life on her own without social support is often an even more difficult alternative.

Many women face another problem. Those who lack English language skills and professional qualifications become trapped in the lower echelons of the job market with no hope of mobility. Deterrents to acquiring English language skills are lack of time, difficulty in following language instruction, and the time of day the classes are held. Although many aspire to fluency in English and better jobs, few are able to achieve either. Many of the sources of distress for these women, then, arise out of the socio-economic circumstances of their lives, and should not be ascribed solely to their cultural or ethnic backgrounds.

Women who are not in the labour force can also have difficulties in

Canada, especially after they have raised their children. Some feel a loss of purpose after the children have left home. Furthermore, they have a sense that housework is not valued in Canadian society. Many feel socially isolated, especially if they lack English language skills.

Another issue facing immigrants pertains to the break up of the family unit as a result of moves to Canada. It is not unusual for one family member to gain entry to Canada, and for relatives and children to follow later. Not only does this pattern of migration disrupt social support networks but family members must also readjust to one another and redefine their family relationships once they are reunited in Canada.

Understanding the dynamics of family life and the importance accorded the family is essential if culturally acceptable, sensitive care is to be provided. Physicians, nurses, social workers, and other health care professionals need to recognize that solutions acceptable to Anglo-Canadian women may be unacceptable to immigrant women. For example, an immigrant woman with an abusive family may flatly refuse to leave her family for fear of being shunned within the ethnic community. Furthermore, "feminist" approaches to the care of a woman may be foreign to her, or may only aggravate her situation. For example, encouraging "assertiveness" and "division of labour" in the home without first understanding the expectations within the particular family may only inflame family feuds and leave the woman as an outsider. Exploring what is acceptable to a woman and what is suited to her situation is crucial for the delivery of effective care. Health professionals need to keep in mind that if a woman loses the support of her family and her ethnic community she may have no one else to turn to because many non-Western, non-English-speaking immigrants are for the most part, marginal in Canadian society.

Influence of the Extended Family on Health Care Decisions

In many immigrant families, the family unit is not only a source of emotional support but it is also an economic unit. Even though the extended family may not live in the same household in Canada, many aspects of extended family life may be carried over. For example, family members may be consulted on important decisions, they may help one another with child care, or with other activities intended to make life in Canada smoother. For many families from Third World countries, obligations and expectations within the family unit are unaltered by geographical separation.

The extended family plays an important part in decision making about help-seeking and illness management. Even though older family members (such as grandparents) may have a weaker position in Canada than in the home country, they may still have a say in health care. Usually, there is deep respect for elders, and their advice about matters relating to health does not go unheeded. For example, it is not uncommon for a grandparent, usually a grandmother, to introduce traditional remedies at the same time that Western medicines are being used. Family members may feel obliged to use them.

Furthermore, grandparents may take over the care of children when a couple goes out to work. They may have to manage a child's illness, and may decide either to use traditional medicine and other traditional health practices, or to combine traditional treatments with Western medicine.

Health professionals also need to keep in mind that although a patient may agree to treatment, he or she may not follow it if the family does not approve. Or, treatment may be adjusted to include the use of traditional remedies. In some instances the dosage may be reduced out of concern that the medication is too strong for the patient.

One of the most trying times for immigrant families in Canada occurs when a family member is hospitalized. Families from many parts of the world expect to be involved in the care of their loved ones. They are used to providing food and attending the sick person in hospital. Unaccustomed to the patterns of health care delivery in this country, many immigrants are concerned that their loved ones will be neglected if they are left alone in hospital. Also, patients expect to have their families with them, otherwise they feel abandoned. Furthermore, being left alone in hospital may be interpreted as loss of family and community.

Many immigrants find hospital personnel lacking in compassion and understanding of the needs of patients and their families. Confronted with hospital rules, many feel helpless, overwhelmed, and alienated from the health care system. Unfortunately these experiences are usually aggravated by language barriers, lack of clear understanding of the disease and treatment procedures, and the stress of having to deal with medical and nursing personnel. While family members may expect to be involved in decisions about the care of their relative, they are usually bewildered by technical language and the overpowering environment of the modern hospital. Patients often feel that their concerns are not taken into account, or that they are being asked to do things that are totally inappropriate. For example, during the postpartum period, a woman may believe that a shower is not only undesirable, but is downright dangerous. Respecting such beliefs would help health professionals to negotiate acceptable care with patients and their families.

Nurses in particular should be aware of the plight of immigrant families and should try to involve them, wherever possible, in a patient's care. Encouraging family members to help by walking the patient or assisting at mealtimes, are only a few of the ways in which family members can be involved. While it may take time before family members understand the explanations, patience will pay off in the end, and health professionals will find both patient and family more co-operative as a result.

Working out a visiting schedule that is acceptable to the nursing staff and the family usually alleviates mutual tensions. While it is recognized that hospital routines demand certain schedules, health professionals and families need to work together to resolve the problems that arise from visiting schedules, and other difficult situations. Understanding what hospitalization means to families, and their need to care for their loved one, is a first step towards providing care that will be perceived as compassionate by the family.

Expectations of Health Professionals

The health care system in Canada is so different from that of most Third World countries that many immigrants and refugees coming from these countries need to be advised about how the system works. For example, many were accustomed to receiving all their care from a clinic, and the idea of having a physician on a long-term basis may be new. The practice of detailed history-taking and lengthy diagnostic procedures may also be foreign, and may be seen as a lack of competence in the physician. Physicians may be expected to know what is wrong and to prescribe medications or other specific treatments promptly.

Many patients are hesitant to ask questions and will appear to agree with what is prescribed. However, this should not be interpreted as real agreement. Rather, many people find it impolite to disagree, and smiling and nodding are simply indications of politeness. It is important to make sure that patients understand the way the system functions, namely that histories are usually taken and tests performed before treatment is prescribed. Furthermore, it should not be assumed that patients will follow treatments, as a variety of factors influence compliance with medical regimens. These include family, beliefs about illness and treatment, and economic factors. Health professionals therefore need to take time to understand the patient's situation and those factors that might influence illness management. While it is important to obtain the patient's story, sensitivity is required so as not to appear intrusive. For example, talking about family relationships may be especially threatening, since respect for family must always be shown, especially to outsiders.

While physicians are highly respected in many Third World countries, nurses do not always have the same prestige. Unlike Canada, in some countries there are few professional schools of nursing, and many nurses receive on-the-job training. They are usually considered as part of the "medical system." Chapter 3 points out that, "nurses . . . should be introduced clearly as professionals to new immigrants. The abilities of nurses and the services they provide, once demonstrated to newcomers, will confirm this status." Many immigrants have reported highly positive interactions with nurses, and quite clearly stereotypes about nursing can be changed once immigrants become aware of the scope of nursing in Canadian society. Nurses who work in community health as well as hospital settings cannot only provide valuable health education and assistance but can also help immigrants to understand the way the health care system works in Canada.

Many immigrants are not familiar with the activities of social workers and may suspect they are acting on behalf of the government. Social work services are usually rare in the immigrant's home country. Interviews aimed at obtaining information about the person's individual situation may be seen as intrusive and a definite threat. Furthermore, people coming from Third World countries may see social services as a last resort, because the use of such services reflects badly on the family. Helping newcomers to understand how these services work is essential if they are to make use of them.

Relationships with Children, and Children in the School System

Although male children are favoured in certain groups, it cannot be assumed that this is always the case. In some groups girls are equally favoured and high value is placed on all children.

To Canadians, some immigrant families may appear overly indulgent of young children. A baby may not be allowed to cry, and may be cuddled either by grandparents, parents, or older siblings. On the other hand, older children may appear to be strictly controlled, as they are expected to show respect for their parents and other family members. Physical punishment, seen as in the child's best interest, may be used in some groups.

Many immigrant families have put their hopes for the future in their children, and a good education is seen as the only way to get ahead. Parents may object to the time the child is expected to spend on non-academic activities. For example, field trips or sports may be seen as not contributing to their goals for the child. Children may be expected to stay home during the evenings to do their homework, instead of socializing with other children. As well, the more liberal aspects of the school curriculum do not always meet with approval from immigrant parents. They may object to the inclusion of sex education, as the discussion of sexual matters may be seen as transgressing the boundaries of good etiquette.

As children become Canadianized, tensions may arise with their parents. Children are usually the first to learn English, and may become interpreters of the outside world for their parents. This gives them a source of power over parents, who become dependent upon them to communicate with authority figures within the larger Canadian society. Health professionals should be aware that using a child as an interpreter can undermine the parents' competence in the eyes of the child. Children should not be used in this capacity, especially when sensitive matters are being discussed.

It is not unheard of for severe communication problems to arise when parents (especially mothers) do not acquire English language skills, and when the child loses the language of the home country. Children who become rapidly socialized into Canadian society may not use their mother tongue outside the home. Communication between mother and child may be diminished if they feel that there is nothing left to talk about. Consequently, parents and children may find that they do not have a common language in which to communicate.

As children learn more about Canadian society, they may object to the forms of discipline used by parents. Whereas physical punishment of a child is seen as normal in some groups, this is not the case in Canada. Parents may be seen as abusive by mainstream Canadians. As children learn about their rights they may report their parents to the authorities. This widens the gulf between children and their families, because parents may see their child as betraying them.

Health professionals should be cautious in their interpretation of what constitutes abuse and should take time to assess the situation carefully. Only by being aware of the problems that can arise from acculturation into a new society can care be given that is appropriate to the family's needs. Health professionals also need to be aware that a child is often caught between two value systems. There is peer pressure to conform to the values of the mainstream group while, on the other hand, the parents may wish the child to follow the values of the home country. Issues arising from dating, especially in the case of female children, may be worrisome for parents, as they may view North American standards as totally unacceptable for their child. This can lead to depression and rebellion, particularly among teenagers.

It must be remembered that the immigrant child needs the support of the family, and every effort should be made to help the parents and child reconcile their differences. Solutions like leaving home, seen as an appropriate measure in some Anglo-Canadian families, may be devastating to an immigrant teenager, who is caught between two worlds. Maintaining ties with a stable ethnic community may, in the long run, serve the child's best interests.

A fairly frequent problem confronting many immigrant families in Canada is that children are sometimes mistakenly assessed as lacking the academic competence to succeed at school. Teachers and health professionals may underestimate the ability of a child who may not be as assertive as children from the mainstream society. Language difficulties and accents may be incorrectly interpreted as incompetence. Extreme sensitivity and understanding is needed in the assessment of children so that they are not channelled into vocational training when they have the talent to succeed in academic programs. Health professionals and teachers need to work collaboratively to identify when a child's apparent learning problems are associated with uprooting and resettlement.

Relationships with Elderly Family Members

The traditionally dominant position of elders may be weakened when they come to Canada as they may become dependent on the children who sponsored them. The fact that older parents are sponsored by their children is sometimes viewed as a threat since young people could potentially withhold support. Elderly parents usually inherit household chores but lose control of the household. This is contrary to the practice in the home country, where elderly family members remain in control of the household but are not expected to do household chores.

One of the most pressing problems for elderly immigrants in Canada is that of social isolation. Many have left their peers behind, and now stay at home to look after their grandchildren. Unaccustomed to the way of life and the transportation system and lacking English, many are afraid to venture out on their own. The lack of English also bars them from using the resources available to other senior citizens.

In addition to the problems of adjusting to a new environment many find that there are conflicts with the younger generation. Their points of view may differ about how the routines of everyday life should be managed or how grandchildren should be raised. But perhaps the most worrisome fact for seniors is that children may be unable to care for them in the home in their old age, as both the women and men in the family may have to go out to work. To be placed in an institution may be unacceptable and interpreted as abandonment. Children, in turn, may feel guilty that they are unable to meet obligations to their parents. Health professionals need to be aware that placement in an institution is not always by choice. Both the elderly and their offspring may need help working through feelings of guilt, resentment, abandonment, and depression.

GUIDELINES FOR CLINICAL PRACTICE

The main issues identified throughout the book provide the basis for the development of guidelines for clinical practice. In this section, the main considerations in assessing patients from different ethnocultural groups will be outlined. Each area of assessment is not meant to mirror particular topics in the preceding section of this chapter. Rather, the suggested questions should yield information that cuts across a number of areas.

Beyond identifying areas for assessment, the *process* of assessment will be discussed, as the kind of data obtained will depend not only on the questions themselves but also on how and when they are asked.

Areas of Assessment

Recognizing the Influence of One's Own Ethnicity and Culture
In western Canada many health professionals are from the mainstream culture. Those who come from a cultural minority group are usually from the upper and middle class and may be unaware of the part their own ethnicity and socio-economic background play in the clinical context. However, not only do health professionals have a "biomedical culture" that is reflected in their work, but also their personal beliefs and values affect their interactions with patients. Patient evaluation, problem definition, and the formulation of possible solutions are not derived solely from impersonal, objective, scientific criteria.

A first step in assessing a patient, therefore, is to recognize one's own ethnicity and social background, and to determine how personal values influence interactions with the patient. Areas of conflict between the values of the health professional and patient have to be acknowledged. For example, in working with women from Third World countries, nurses and physicians need to realize that their own values may influence their interpretation of a woman's situation and solutions that they consider appropriate. Health professionals who value assertiveness may be frustrated by what they perceive to be a woman's passivity.

The values of the health professional are not just personal but may reflect values in the work environment and the societal context. For example, performing tasks efficiently, with little social conversation and time with the patient, may be thought to exemplify a good doctor. Similarly, hospital nurses may see the efficient discharge of tasks as more important than taking time to assess the patient's and family's situation.

Even where health professional and patient come from the same ethnic background they will not necessarily share similar beliefs and values. In fact, Kleinman (1986) has noted that social factors like gender, class, education, and occupational differences may outweigh shared cultural origins. He points out that, "even when ethnicity is the same, practitioners need to evaluate how class, religious affiliation, gender, age and other differences may make it particularly difficult for them to work with their own patients" (p. 4). In many instances physicians coming from Third World countries are from the upper classes, and therefore class differences are quite likely to exist between them and many of the patients from their homelands.

Establishing the Role of the Patient's Ethnicity in Beliefs about Illness
Many factors make for intra-ethnic diversity; it cannot be assumed that individuals will always subscribe to commonly held beliefs about health and illness. A second step in assessment is to establish the role that the patient's ethnicity plays in experiences of illness, health beliefs, and practices. To avoid ethnic stereotyping, the pattern of questioning in an initial interview should be directed at locating the patient's ethnic and social position. Questions should be handled so as to put the patient at ease. Examples of questions that will help the health professional to obtain a sense of the kind of patient being dealt with include:
- place of birth (if not in Canada, find out if in a city or in the country);
- length of time in Canada and whether the patient had family in this country before arriving;
- kind of job in the home country; and

– kind of job in Canada.

Ascertaining this information will shed light on the patient's background and a number of other pertinent issues. If the patient is an urban professional, there will quite likely be greater familiarity with Western medicine than is the case with patients from rural farming backgrounds. The patient's occupation in Canada may also alert the health professional to downward socio-economic mobility and difficulty in adjusting to life in Canada.

Questions about level of education, although useful in placing a patient, can be humiliating for those with little schooling. The clinician has to decide when the timing is appropriate.

Professionals need to establish the kinds of medical systems patients have encountered in the past. Everyone coming into Canada will have had some contact with Western medicine for purposes of immigration, but many might have used the traditional medicine of their homelands. Where patients are more familiar with traditional medicine, it is necessary to find out more about these beliefs and practices, and to identify where they conflict with the professional's understandings, plans, and expectations.

The process of assessment continues over time. Many people are reluctant to reveal their beliefs and health practices to strangers. More time will have to be spent on patients who are reticent.

Determining Differences in Viewpoints of Patients and Clinicians about Health and Illness

Health professionals and patients quite often bring different notions to the clinical encounter. Professionals bring their biomedical culture as well as beliefs and values derived from their ethnic and socio-cultural background. Patients bring their interpretation of the biomedical model, and a set of beliefs and values about illness. There may be, and often are, discrepancies between these two perspectives in the explanation of disease and illness, the expectations of how each should behave, and of treatment results. These discrepancies exist even where patients and professionals come from the mainstream culture. When the patient is from a traditional background the likelihood of mutual discrepancy is much greater.

Health professionals must consciously find out the extent to which their own viewpoints differ from those of their patients. The issue here is not that viewpoints differ, but that these differences can lead to misunderstanding and affect the results of treatment. Health professionals therefore need to explore with patients their beliefs about illness, expectations of treatment, and how illness is managed in daily life.

We noted earlier that patients are sometimes hesitant to discuss their beliefs for fear of being ridiculed. Furthermore, many do not expect to be questioned about their views; they believe the physician should know what is wrong with them without excessive questioning. Timing is important in introducing questions; sensitivity is also needed in phrasing questions which should not be judgmental. The line of questioning suggested here is not meant as a rigid prescription for a first interview. Rather, these are areas to be covered— quite likely over several interviews. Patients may discuss their beliefs about illness only after they are convinced of the health professional's competence. Treatments of some sort may have to be prescribed simply to demonstrate to the patient that the physician knows what is wrong.

The following questions suggested by Kleinman (1980) and used by some physicians and nurses in clinical practice, have been found to be helpful in obtaining data about patients' understanding of their illness. These questions are:

1 What do you call your problem? What name do you give it?
2 What do you think has caused it?
3 Why did it start when it did?
4 What does your sickness do to your body? How does it work inside you?
5 How severe is it? Will it get better soon or take longer?
6 What do you fear most about your sickness?
7 What are the chief problems your sickness has caused for you (personally, in your family, and at work)?
8 What kind of treatment do you think you should receive? What are the most important results you hope you will receive from the treatment? (Kleinman 1980, 1986)

In addition, information should be obtained about the home remedies used. Such areas should include:

1 the kinds of home remedies people use for this illness;
2 home remedies that are currently being used and that are judged to be helpful; and
3 remedies used in the past and their effectiveness.

Kleinman cautions that the proposed questions should not be presented as a list to the patient. Both the timing and phrasing of questions should be adapted to the individual. That is, the questions are interwoven into the interview and are asked only when the clinician senses that their introduction is appropriate. In other words, the questions are not posed in isolation from the rest of an interview. They should be asked in such a way as to demonstrate the health professional's genuine interest in what the patient has to say.

Identifying the Influence of the Family on Health Care and Identifying Social Support Networks

Family members play an important part in health care decisions, especially when illness is managed in the home. The likelihood that a patient will follow prescribed treatments often depends on how they are viewed by the family. Certain key people in the family may have the final say. It is important to find out who these people are.

Another factor should be kept in mind by health professionals. The proximity of numerous relatives does not always mean that the patient feels supported by the family. In fact, tensions within a family can encourage isolation and loneliness in individual family members, even when there are several members in a household. In addition to the ups and downs of everyday life, beliefs about a particular illness and its cultural meaning, may have a profound impact on the kind of support the sick person receives. Finding out about the structure and functioning of the family is therefore critical. The following areas should be included in the assessment:

- marital status;
- presence of extended family in household (grandmothers, grandfathers, older aunts and uncles, etc.);
- relatives in the local community;
- kinds of home remedies used in the home country—and whether they are used in this country;
- children in the family (starting with questions about children, especially when interviewing mothers, usually puts people at ease). Find out how children are doing in school and at home;
- support: inside and outside the home; if woman works, who helps at home;
- who the person turns to for help and the kinds of help that are sought; and
- elderly family members—find out how they are managing.

Questions about family life should be approached with caution. Many immigrants consider family life and problems as personal, and regard questions on the subject as intrusive. The health professional may be wise to await a cue from the patient that the time is ripe.

Establishing if there are Difficulties in Adjustment

Uprooting from one's home country and settling in a new country are traumatic under the best of circumstances. Coupled with this, most immigrants have to find employment, cope with language problems, and manage on a tight budget. How a patient experiences and manages illness may be inextricably linked to the issues surrounding adjustment. Therefore, it is imperative that health professionals establish if there are difficulties in adjustment. Areas to explore include:

- employment status—kind of job. Establish if there is downward mobility for both men and women;
- English language skills—assessed from moment of first contact, but the patient may discuss problems of proficiency in getting a well-paid job;
- gender-related issues (might also surface under family life);
- trouble with adolescent children;
- financial support: how family is currently obtaining income; and
- how the cost of health care is currently being paid.

Tact is needed in posing these questions so that the patient will not feel threatened. These are obviously not the areas to explore early in the relationship. Patients usually give cues when they feel sufficiently at ease to discuss such matters with a physician or nurse.

In addition, physical examinations and other diagnostic procedures are usually required to complete the assessment of a patient. Consideration has to be given to cultural variations in executing these procedures. For example, women coming from some countries may be reluctant to be examined by a male physician or be cared for by a male nurse and older male patients may object to being examined by a young female physician. Sensitivity is required in dealing with these issues to ensure that the patient is not humiliated.

As well, some diagnostic procedures may be refused. For example, a patient may refuse to give blood as the loss of blood may be seen to weaken and harm the body. It is important for health professionals to understand the patient's system of beliefs and not to interpret the patient's behaviour as non-compliance.

THE PROCESS OF ASSESSMENT

Assessment is a clinical art that combines sensitivity, clinical judgment, and scientific knowledge. Not only must one know when to ask questions, but also how to phrase them so that the patient does not find them offensive. The clinician should be alert to data that can be elicited without direct questioning. Yet there is also the need to guard against premature conclusions. Observations should be validated to avoid making incorrect assumptions. For example, if a woman wears traditional dress it should not be assumed that she subscribes to traditional medical practices. In the course of the interview, data should be obtained to reach a valid conclusion about her health beliefs and practices.

The process of assessment goes on over time. While certain data have to be obtained in an initial interview so as to deal with pressing medical or nursing problems, patients should not be expected to share sensitive information until trust has been established. Patients may also be reluctant to discuss the use of herbal remedies. Direct questioning, such as "Are you using herbal remedies?" in the early stages of a relationship may be seen as intrusive and lead only to denial.

Once trust has been built information might be shared quite spontaneously, especially if the patient is concerned about the efficacy of a traditional remedy and if it is being used solely because of family pressure. In fact, a community health nurse recalled an experience with a patient who had elected to use herbal remedies instead of Western medicine. This information was volunteered by the patient, but only after several visits to the patient's home. Health professionals can facilitate this process by asking questions phrased in a non-judgmental way, for example, "Have you found anything else that has helped you?" This kind of question might be more acceptable than, "Are you taking other medicines besides those prescribed by the doctor?"

Similarly, patients may be reluctant to reveal traditional beliefs about illness to the Western health professional for fear of being ridiculed. The timing of such questions is important and professionals have to rely on their clinical judgment about when such questions should be asked. Furthermore, health professionals should be aware that some patients expect them to know immediately what is wrong and what treatment is appropriate. Thus, questions like, "What do you think has caused your illness?" or "What kind of treatment do you think you should receive?" if asked at the wrong time and in the wrong context, may only bewilder the patient. Clinical abilities may have to be demonstrated before such questions can be asked!

A common problem is that the patient does not have English language competence. In such instances it is essential to use an interpreter. Yet using an interpreter is not without difficulty. For example, the interpreter may give a précis of what the patient says, grossly altering the meaning of the communication. The clinician should be sure to ask the interpreter to translate verbatim. Another problem is that the interpreter and patient may be from a different social class. The interpreter may be embarrassed to discuss folk beliefs, wanting instead to portray the culture in a certain light. Therefore, the interpreter should know the clinician is genuinely interested in the patient's viewpoint, sees it as legitimate, and as an essential part of the treatment plan. The use of family members as interpreters often inhibits frankness in patients. For reasons mentioned earlier, children should not be used to interpret for their parents.

A small point, but worth mentioning, is that the dialogue should be between the clinician and the patient—the interpreter translates in the background as it were. This facilitates the building of rapport with the patient even if there is not a common language.

ACCOMMODATING THE PATIENT'S VIEWPOINT AND NEGOTIATING APPROPRIATE CARE

Patients from different ethnic groups and class backgrounds have different expectations of their encounters with health professionals, physicians in particular. Some patients expect that the physician will diagnose their illness and prescribe treatment. They do not expect to be, nor do they want to be, equal partners in the dialogue. Others want to be actively involved in the treatment process.

Passivity in the clinical encounter does not imply acceptance of the prescribed treatment regimen. Patients usually have notions about appropriate ways of interacting with health professionals. Doctors, for the most part, are seen as authority figures to be respected. Passivity is a demonstration of respect. Once they are in their own homes, however, patients may use alternative healing practices concurrently with Western medications. Or, they may modify the medication dosage, if they believe that the Western medicine is too strong. They may even elect not to use the Western medicine. These practices, for obvious reasons, are usually not admitted to physicians and nurses. The physician and nurse therefore must consciously find out about illness management. It should be clear to patients that the intent is not to judge these practices, but to assist in the effective management of an illness.

Finding out what the patient believes and the treatment plan that the patient follows (which may be different from that prescribed by the clinician) is preparatory to working out mutually acceptable, yet effective ways for treating the patient. For example, the physician or nurse may find out that some families use traditional remedies in addition to the prescribed biomedicine. Sometimes this might be perfectly acceptable, as the use of both types of treatment poses no risk to the patient. In treating some illnesses, however, there might be substantial risk to the patient if traditional and Western treatments are combined. It is in instances such as these that ways must be found to negotiate appropriate care with the patient.

While the process of negotiation is usually one in which the patient and health professional present their viewpoints and work out a mutually satisfying solution, some patients might not expect this conduct in their encounters with health professionals. If requested to interact with professionals in this way, it is quite possible that they will become bewildered and doubtful about the expertise of the clinician. Rather, in most instances, negotiation occurs when there are conflicts in treatment practices, and where these practices may be harmful to the well-being of the patient. For example, replacing insulin therapy with herbal remedies, or varying medication dosages, may be detrimental to a patient. These are the issues that become critical in the process of negotiation.

One cannot devise a recipe for negotiating with a patient. Each situation will be different. Often, however, the clinician has to find out precisely how the patient is managing the illness and what practices could be harmful. This should be done in a non-judgmental way. The clinician has to decide what aspects of the patient's remedies can safely be combined with Western medicine. In such instances, both traditional and Western remedies may be used concurrently. When the patient reduces dosages for fear that the medication is too strong, the physician has to decide if the patient can get by on the reduced dosage. In those instances when harm might result, the patient should know what the possible outcome might be. Trying to reach a compromise about treatment will sometimes involve other family members, who often have a strong influence on the patient.

Negotiation takes many forms. It may involve frank and open exchange of ideas, gentle persuasion, debate, disagreement, or confrontation. It can also demand interpretation of, and response to, non-verbal cues as the sole form of communication. Or communication may be through a third party. Progress towards resolution may be immediate or may fluctuate over months or even years.

The following case history demonstrates one form that negotiation can take.

Case History: Chinese Family with a Premature Infant

During the first week at home both the mother, who was unwell, and baby, who was having difficulty sucking, required several visits by the community health nurse accompanied by an interpreter. The young mother asked her visiting mother-in-law, who was assisting with the care of the baby, to show the nurse the herbal preparation she was giving the infant. While the grandmother was showing the bottle to the interpreter the mother gestured frantically to the nurse, indicating that she did not want the baby to have the mixture. The nurse asked the interpreter to have the grandmother tell her about the herb, how she had used it in China, and to describe what she valued about it. The next step involved detailed explanation of the characteristics of premature babies and their need for close monitoring to promote stability and growth. Since neither the nurse nor the interpreter recognized the herbal mixture, the nurse asked the grandmother if she would consider waiting until the baby was a bit bigger before adding it to the present breast and bottle program. She agreed and the mother expressed relief and gratitude.

In this instance, the nurse had to negotiate with the grandmother so that the treatment regimen for the child could be effected. It is not unusual for grandmothers (from a variety of cultures) to have considerable say during the prenatal and postnatal periods. Child-rearing and child-bearing are often regarded as their area of expertise and they may question Western practices. In fact, they may correctly argue that their methods have worked over many generations. In instances such as these the professional has to determine what is in the best interest of the mother and child. Skillful interpersonal interactions will be required to work with the grandmother to reach a satisfactory compromise.

In some instances a patient may elect to follow the culturally specific treatment practices and might refuse all prescribed medical or nursing treatment. In these situations the goal becomes one of monitoring the patient's condition in order to identify changes in health state and recognize impending crises before they become irreversible. On occasion, the reality of crisis and impending loss of health and function provides the opportunity to renegotiate the care approach.

It is important that patients are not rejected for non-compliance and that assistance is continued to maintain the optimal level of health under the circumstances. In addition, it is crucial that regardless of the individual's final decision about a care or treatment, relationships with the health professional remain on a positive note. Otherwise, future success with the individual or family members will be unlikely.

Of course, there are situations when the patient is not lawfully free to make choices where these are detrimental to others. Two such examples are refusal to accept treatment for tuberculosis and the neglect or abuse of children. In these instances, the health professional is obliged to intervene.

Finally, we must remember that most non-medical and non-Western remedies may indeed have stood the test of time, and may in fact prove to have beneficial effects.

CROSS-CULTURAL CARING EXERCISES

The following cross-cultural vignettes are included as examples of some of the situations that physicians and nurses are required to confront. Consider the kinds of information you would need from patients and their families to make an adequate assessment, then proceed to address the questions.

Vignette 1

A thirty-five-year-old Chinese man comes to the office complaining of stomach pain. On questioning, you discover the pain is non-specific and intermittent, and localized to the epigastrium. He came from mainland China three months ago.
- What would you want to know about his life circumstance and background?
- What special meaning may be attached to "stomach pain" by this man?
- What treatments may he have tried?
- How may your diagnosis or management be influenced by his cultural origin?

Vignette 2

A couple from Libya has come to see you because the woman is pregnant. The husband tells you that his wife is not eating properly and that he wants her in the hospital. The wife wears traditional dress and does not speak.
- How would you proceed with the assessment?
- With whom do you negotiate? Husband? Wife? Both?
- What is the implication of her "not eating" to the husband? To the wife?
- What are their fears?
- How will you decide whether hospitalization is necessary?

Vignette 3

The breast-feeding wife of a student from India comes to see you with her new baby, accompanied by her mother-in-law. The baby's weight gain is low, according to the standard growth curve.
- Who do you tell?
- What do you say?
- What are the risks in communicating the information and formulating a management plan?

Vignette 4

A young man, a recent immigrant from Uganda, complains to you of night sweats and weight loss.
- What conditions do you consider in your preliminary diagnostic formulation?
- What bearing does his country of origin have?
- What is his understanding of or concern about the symptoms?

FURTHER READING

Anderson, Joan M. "The cultural context of caring," *Canadian Critical Care Nursing Journal*, Vol. 4, No. 4 (1987):7–13

Caring across Cultures: Multicultural Considerations in Palliative Care. Prepared by St. Elizabeth Visiting Nurses' Association of Ontario, Palliative Care Support Team 1988

Kleinman, A. *Patients and Healers in the Context of Culture*. Berkeley, CA: University of California Press 1980

--. "Culture in the Clinic: A Clinical Framework for Assessing Cultural Problems in Patient Care," paper presented at the School of Nursing, University of British Columbia 1986

Kleinman, A., L. Eisenberg, and B. Good. "Culture, Illness, and Care," *Annals of Internal Medicine*, Vol. 88 (1978): 251-58

Immigration Regulations and Provision of Health Services to Immigrants

Danica Gleave

Immigrants to Canada have numbered around 90,000 a year since 1980. Roughly half these people enter the country under the Family Class designation, while refugees and people in refugee-like situations make up another group, as do the various types of Independent Immigrants. These classes were outlined in the Immigration Act proclaimed in 1978 and some parts were revised in 1988. Immigration policies and procedures, to a degree, are open to interpretation by the federal government of the day.

FAMILY CLASS

The purpose of this legislative designation is the reunification of families. Immigrants qualifying under this class are in most cases the parents, grandparents, fiancé, spouse, or children of the sponsoring Canadian citizen or Landed Immigrant. The sponsoring family must meet specific income requirements, after which the application is processed abroad in the home country of the prospective immigrant. Family class members are the highest priority of the immigration program (along with refugees) and account for 40 to 50 per cent of the total number of immigrants coming to Canada. Nearly half come from Asia, with Europe providing 20 per cent. Other relatives must come as Assisted Relatives under the Independent Immigrants category (see below).

INDEPENDENT IMMIGRANTS

Any independent immigrant must qualify under one of the following categories, and must acquire sufficient points to be admitted. Having a relative in Canada, knowledge of English and/or French, having a prearranged job, and sound financial status are some of the factors by which a person can win points. The values assigned to these abilities are subject to change.

ASSISTED RELATIVES

Assisted Relatives are family members who do not qualify under Family Class or Independent provisions. These include: brothers and sisters; grandparents; parents; grandchildren; aunts; uncles; nieces and nephews. In all cases a citizen or permanent resident must give a written undertaking to assist the immigrant to come to Canada and become established here. Brothers and sisters account for about three-quarters of all applicants.

ECONOMIC IMMIGRANTS

Newcomers who want to qualify under this heading must be either entrepreneurs, investors, self-employed persons, or retirees who are self-sufficient. Entrepreneurs must establish or purchase a large share of a business which they will help manage and which will employ at least one other Canadian. The investor category created in 1986 is meant to encourage people with $150,000 or more to invest in a Canadian enterprise. Hong Kong followed by Western Europe have been the largest sources of immigrants in the economic groups.

Self-employed persons are admitted with the intention of establishing a business in which they work or contributing to the artistic or cultural life of the country.

Retirees are Independent Immigrants who have completed their working lives and who are admitted on the understanding that they will not become part of the Canadian labour force. They must also guarantee that they are financially capable of meeting their own needs without Canadian government support.

HUMANITARIAN PROGRAMS FOR REFUGEES AND DESIGNATED CLASSES

The category currently most in flux and in the public eye is refugees and people in similar circumstances. Since the mid-1980s they have met differing degrees of welcome when applying to Canada for asylum. The Immigration Act contains provisions for Convention Refugees as defined by the United Nations High Commission on Refugees. These are people who have been forced to flee their homes and countries and who have a well-founded fear of persecution.

Convention Refugees make up about 25 per cent of the people whom Canada accepts in this general group. The remainder are those in refugee-like situations, including the Indochinese (Cambodia, Laos, and Vietnam), political prisoners (from Chile, El Salvador, Guatemala, Poland, and Uruguay) and self-exiled people (mostly from eastern Europe). Canada supports efforts to resettle refugees in areas geographically and culturally close to their original homes, but for many this is not a viable option.

Most potential refugees apply for admission while still in their home country, in a refugee camp, or from a neighbouring country where they are seeking temporary shelter. Some apply directly at the Canadian border or from within Canada once they arrive. Examples of the latter include Central Americans who have walked northwards or Sri Lankans who make claims after arriving at an airport. Each approach results in different bureaucratic procedures.

Potential refugees whose applications from abroad are accepted can come to Canada secure in the knowledge that they have been granted permanent resident status (also called landed immigrant status). They are entitled to federal assistance, in the form of travel loans, five months of language training in English or French, one year of medical coverage, and assistance with housing and other expenses. After waiting three years, they can apply for citizenship like any other landed immigrant. The major drawback is that not every refugee claimant is able to remain in safety near the Canadian embassy where they have applied, for the several months required to process the claim.

For those claimants coming directly to the border or airport, the procedure is similar except that, until recently, the waiting period prior to acceptance sometimes lasted many months or even years. A new set of procedures, made into law in 1988, was designed to shorten the waiting period and to ensure that those who were transporting people to Canada under false pretenses were discouraged. Now, a person arriving at the border or airport must state his or her intent to claim refugee status and must then wait for an initial hearing before an adjudicator. At some times this hearing has been delayed for several weeks. If the person's refugee claim is judged valid the second step of the process requires appearance before a two-member board that accepts or rejects the claim. Although the new policy is designed to greatly reduce the claimant's waiting period, there are still some persons who must wait several months for a decision. A small proportion of refugee claims have been rejected and the person thus sent out of Canada, sometimes back to the home country. During this period of limbo between filing the claim and the final decision minimal support for food and rent is available. However, claimants do not qualify for subsidized language training, health insurance (except in emergencies), education, or free legal assistance, and they cannot sponsor family members (spouses, children) who were left behind.

If a claim is refused, applicants may appeal to the Federal Court of Appeal and remain in Canada while they do so. Most do not have the financial means to do that.

All refugee claimants must pass a physical examination as part of the screening process. Handicapped claimants must obtain prior approval from their admitting province before they will be accepted.

Non-governmental organizations such as churches and community groups sponsor about one-quarter of all refugees in Canada, providing newcomers with furniture, clothing, language training, and so on. Most importantly, they provide a community of support for people who have been displaced.

Between 1980 and 1985 western Canada provided new homes to 45,000 refugees who were ultimately accepted as permanent residents. It is also worth noting that in 1986 Canada was awarded the Nansen Medal by the United Nations in recognition of the work it has done in resettling refugees.

GENERAL NOTES ON MEDICAL COVERAGE

Provincial policies vary, but in British Columbia only Canadian citizens, landed immigrants, and those who are in Canada under employment and student authorization qualify for services under the Medical Services Plan. People must have been residents of the province for at least three months before they are eligible for coverage. For wealthy immigrants who can afford private health insurance this poses little problem. For others, it can be a major problem. Refugee claimants and illegal immigrants are not entitled to Medical Services coverage.

FURTHER READING

Employment and Immigration Canada. *Canada's Immigration Law*. Ottawa: Ministry of Supply and Services 1989
—. *Claiming Refugee Status in Canada*. Ottawa: Ministry of Supply and Services 1989